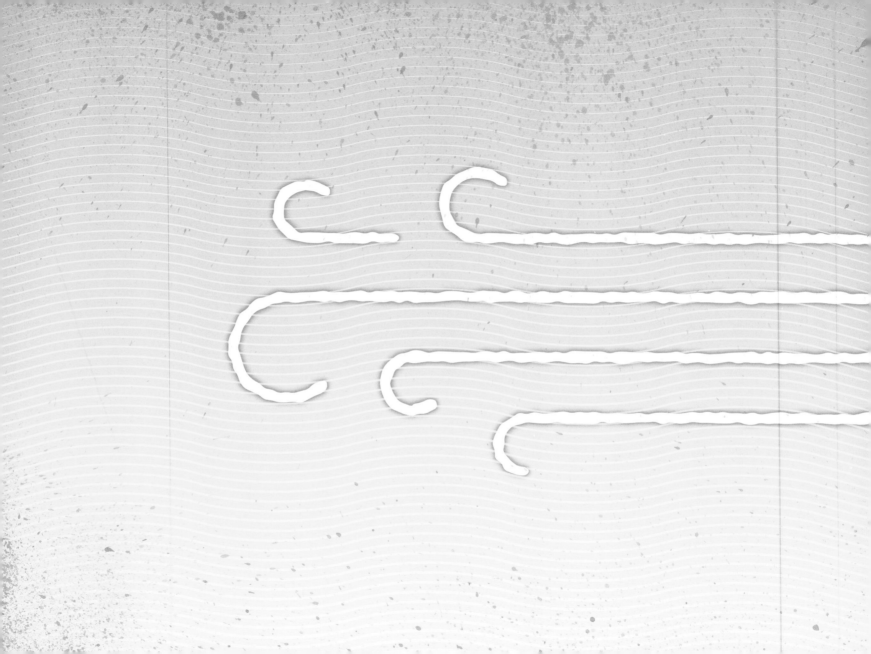

foreword by
**Vidyamala Burch
& Anna Black**

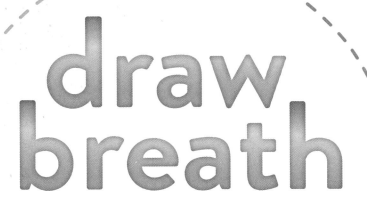

draw
breath

THE ART OF BREATHING,
MINDFULNESS &
MEDITATION

TOM GRANGER

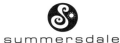

summersdale

An Hachette UK Company

www.hachette.co.uk

Summersdale Publishers Ltd
Part of Octopus Publishing Group Limited
Carmelite House
50 Victoria Embankment
LONDON
EC4Y 0DZ
UK
www.summersdale.com

Printed and bound in China

ISBN: 978-1-78783-033-2

Substantial discounts on bulk quantities of Summersdale books are available to corporations, professional associations and other organizations. For details contact general enquiries: telephone: **+44 (0) 1243 771107** or email: **enquiries@summersdale.com.**

For my greatest heroes,

Melanie and John

Health information and disclaimer – please read before engaging in the practices

Every effort has been made to ensure that the information in this book is accurate and current at the time of publication. The author and the publisher cannot accept responsibility for any misuse or misunderstanding of any information contained herein, or any loss, damage or injury, be it health, financial or otherwise, suffered by any individual or group acting upon or relying on information contained herein.

None of the opinions or suggestions in this book is intended to replace medical opinion. This book is about conscious breathing and suggests breathing techniques. This is not medical advice and does not take the place of such advice. If you have concerns about your health, please seek professional advice. If you have any medical conditions you should consult a medical practitioner before you follow any techniques in this book. Please do not practice any of these exercises while driving or handling heavy machinery.

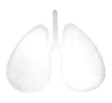

BODY

Here we delve into the anatomy of the breath and learn some simple breathing techniques that can be used to fundamentally alter our physiology and balance our internal states. We will begin to investigate how the movement of our bodies affects the world of our emotions.

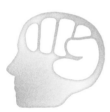

MIND

In this section we explore some of the philosophy behind conscious, mindful breathing, learning how it can be used to strengthen our mental focus and make us more calm, resilient and creative. We will also take a look at how small shifts in perspective can change our world view on a larger scale.

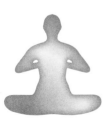

SPIRIT

Finally, we learn how we can use our new skills in "hacking" our physiology and consciousness to live and appreciate a more rewarding life, for ourselves and those around us. Shifting our focus from breathing to drawing, we will use art as a tool for learning about the nature of perception and see how drawing from life can become a transcendent experience.

Don't jump ahead... yet!

The exercises are designed to be completed from front to back with each building on the previous and informing the next.

For best results, start at the beginning of the book and work your way through. While it will probably be tempting to jump ahead to an image or project that stands out to you, I urge you to take your time and build up to the exercises that come later in the book. This is particularly true for the image tracing tasks near the back of the book and the longer breathing practices.

Once you are around a third of the way through the book, you will have the basics covered. At this point, feel free to ignore the chronology and carry out the practices that jump out at you.

It is important that you read the instructions for each individual practice to get the most out of it... every exercise is subtly different.

You will notice that there is subtle overlap between the sections; this is because all of the elements are connected. Conscious breathing enhances the connection between body and mind; by realizing and experiencing that they are one system, we enlighten the spirit.

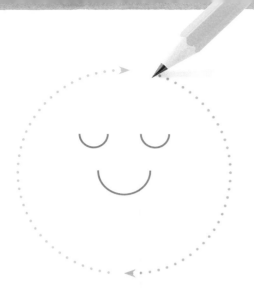

FOREWORD BY VIDYAMALA BURCH

When I first opened *Draw Breath* I was captivated. Gazing at a page evoked a kind of silence and space that was immediately calming. When I dived deeper and embarked on the journey the book offers, I knew I had something special in my hands.

The modern world can be a very noisy place to live. From dawn to dusk we are bombarded with words, sounds, phone calls, text messages, social media, 24-hour news channels. The omnipresent buzz of life can, at times, seem overwhelming. Our senses are so overloaded that it can be hard to find any respite and our nervous systems become continually aroused and hyper-stimulated.

This is one of the reasons so many of us are unhappy and exhausted. We are "switched on" for too many hours of the day and the natural human longing and need for peace seems a far-off dream.

If we are to be well, individually and collectively, we need to consciously find ways to cultivate calm and ease. We need to learn how to reset our nervous systems so we can unwind and recharge and return to some kind of balance.

Put simply, we need to give ourselves space to breathe. Literally. In and out. Rhythmically and smoothly.

We can write about the benefits of mindful breathing. We can talk about it. We can explore concepts around it. We can issue exhortations to notice defensive patterns of breath-holding and to let go – to let the out-breath find its full expression as it sighs to its conclusion. But these are just *more words* in a world already drowning in words. It is unlikely that they will have much impact.

Tom knows this and he uses words sparingly and brilliantly whilst conveying deep, profound ideas with images, aesthetics and drawing exercises. Rather than reading about healthy breathing you'll find yourself tasting it as soon as you complete one of the exercises. Your breathing will slow. Your mind will change. Your emotions will become more spacious and creative. You'll need no convincing of the power of breath-awareness because you will have had an embodied experience of learning – always the most powerful and lasting way to embed new perspectives.

Tom also has a great skill for "word play". Through double-meaning the literal mind is tricked away from habitual, superficial understanding. Tom's use of language becomes a gateway to deeper truths. From the title *"Draw Breath"* to the very last page of the book, I noticed my mind flexing to re-visit the meaning of common words and in doing so it was startled into amazement and wonder.

I love this book. I love plunging beneath a sea of words to rest in something much deeper. I love the way Tom knows that this is what so many of us need, and he has the talent and ability to bring this experience (I hesitate to call it a book) into being. Savour it and enjoy it. Your nervous system and mind will be grateful. They will, quite simply, thank you for taking the time to breathe.

Vidyamala Burch

Vidyamala sustained a spinal injury when she was 16. Over 25 years ago she started exploring mindfulness and meditation to manage her persistent pain. In 2001 she co-founded Breathworks based on all she had learned and it has since grown into the UK's largest and most well-respected mindfulness teacher training organization. She has been a practicing Buddhist for many years and was ordained into the Triratna Buddhist Order in 1995. In 2008 she published *Living Well with Pain and Illness* (Piatkus), and in 2013 she co-authored *You Are Not Your Pain* (titled *Mindfulness for Health* in the UK) (Piatkus). Both these books are based on the Breathworks approach.

www.breathworks-mindfulness.org.uk
www.vidyamala-burch.com

FOREWORD BY ANNA BLACK

In my own work as an artist and as a teacher of both mindfulness meditation and Betty Edwards's Drawing on the Right Side of the Brain® course, I've always been interested in the links between drawing and meditation. Experiencing that place where "I" gets out of the way, the critical voice shuts up and all there is is the moment of the mark appearing as the drawing draws itself. That is when the *magic* happens.

Too often, though, we get caught up in an unhelpful cycle of judgement and expectations about how we *think* our drawing is *supposed* to be. The same thing can happen when we meditate: our mind, crammed full of monkeys having a bun fight, is judged a "bad" practice; or the monkeys are snoozing so that must be a "good" one. The reality is, whether your monkey mind is having a party or taking time out, the invitation is always just to notice how it is, and let go of wanting things to be a particular way.

When we can allow things to be as they are, we are no longer resisting our experience and a myriad of possibilities can arise.

I love *Draw Breath* because it encourages you to simply *be* with your experience and the process of mark-making. There is no right or wrong or an expectation to produce something that another will judge as "a good drawing". Your breath is unique and every exploration you make of it will be too.

Draw Breath is a practice you can come back to time and time again. There's no need to try and categorize or label it. You may enjoy some exercises more than others; you may get bored, frustrated, or feel calm or relaxed. Tom's invitation is simply to explore and discover your breath, what it has to tell you and how you relate to that. Enjoy the journey!

Anna Black

Anna Black has been teaching mindfulness meditation since 2006. She has written numerous books on mindfulness including *Living in the Moment* (2012, Cico Books) and *Mindfulness on the Go* book and card set (2017, Cico Books). Her books have been translated into six languages. Anna is also an artist and a certified and licensed Drawing on the Right Side of the Brain® teacher. She has been teaching Drawing on the Right Side of the Brain® workshops in the UK since 2008. She brings drawing and meditation together in her Mindful Drawing workshops, which she has been running since 2014.

www.mindfulness-meditation-now.com
www.learn-to-draw-right.com
www.annalouisablack.com

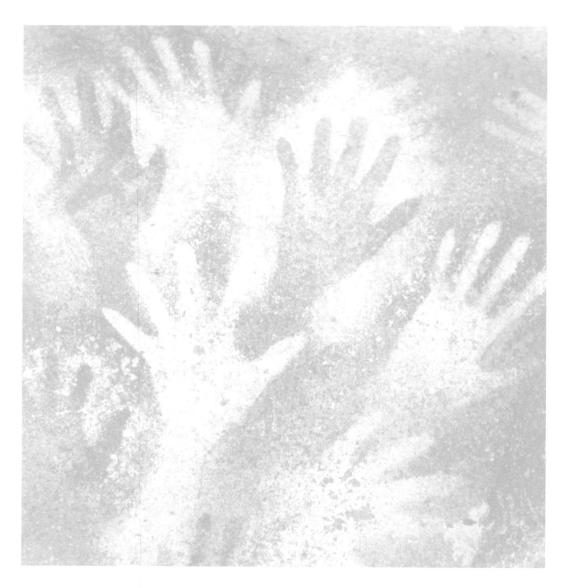

The art of breathing

From the remote islands of Indonesia to the deep caves of Northern Europe, and all the way to the tip of South America, the same motif can be found: a human hand. Reaching out of history, these handprints chart the odyssey of our ancestors as *Homo sapiens* traversed the globe. At 40,000 years old, they are the earliest evidence of human beings creating art.

It is their humanity and simplicity that make these images so enduringly compelling. It's easy to imagine putting your own hand over the imprint of your distant relative, contemplating who they may have been and why they made these marks.

While there are many theories as to *why* these marks were made, there is no doubt as to *how*. The first artist created these impressions by grinding mineral oxides into powder and putting this pigment into their mouth to mix with their saliva and form paint. With short, powerful breaths, they blew it through a pipe made of bone or wood over their hand as they pressed it against the cave wall.

Forty millennia before Banksy, human beings were using their own breath as a spray can and their own bodies as a stencil, creating beautiful graffiti that remains stunning to this day.

To us, this Palaeolithic artwork appears to say, *"We were here"*, but to the artists, whether they were shamans conducting spiritual ceremonies or simply families entertaining their children, this was a deliberate, visceral, full-body process that, in one way or another, said, *"We are here."* They were using their own bodies as medium, subject and, quite possibly, meaning.

Draw Breath aims to use your breath, your body and your innate creativity to make simple art to a similar end. Art doesn't have to mean something big to have a big meaning. Just like when you inhale deeply, exhale noisily onto the cold bathroom mirror and use your finger to squeakily scrawl a message to a loved one, it is often the simplest, in-the-moment creations that are the most honest and elating.

It is my sincere wish that through the simple meditative tasks in this book you may connect deeply to your breath, and through it, enhance your connection between your own body and mind. At the very least, I hope that somewhere in these pages you experience a few moments of peace and relaxation in your busy life.

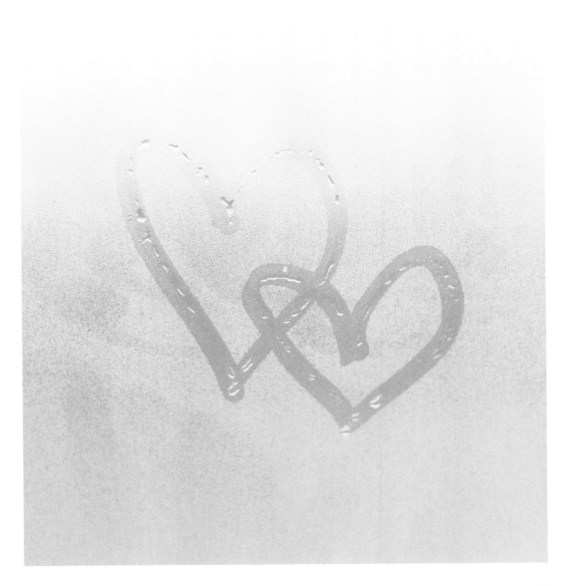

Drawing as meditation

When students are taught Japanese calligraphy, often one of the first symbols they learn is *"ensō"* – the circle.

The *ensō* is drenched in figurative meaning yet remains deliberately ambiguous in pictorial power. The true meaning of the *ensō* is difficult to translate, not from Japanese into English but from a symbol into words.

Depending on which Zen master you ask, they will tell you that it represents everything, or it represents nothing, or, more likely, that it represents both. It depicts the cycle of birth and death, the sun, the moon, the universe, the inside, the outside, completeness, harmony, infinity, even enlightenment.

Ensō as a concept represents many things, but an individual *ensō* depicts a moment in time for the artist who draws it...

... a single, deliberate movement, committed to paper with a clear mind, in time with the body's natural exhalation.

The resulting art is the record of a process. A mental and physical experience, expressed in ink. It can be measured by its honesty, its vitality and the beauty of its imperfections.

It is from this philosophy that *Draw Breath* takes its inspiration... Each exercise in this book will ask you to make an honest record of your breath and notice its effects on your body and your consciousness.

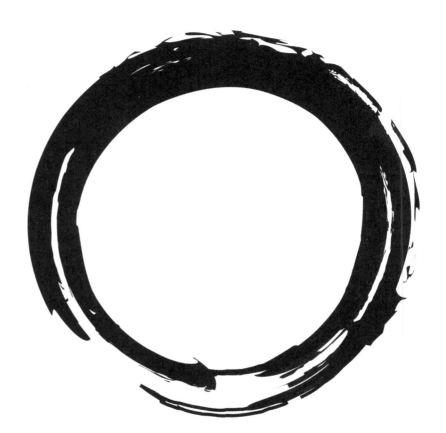

"ensō"

Why focus on breathing?

We can go without food for more than a month. We can last without sleep for almost a fortnight. We can live without water for a couple of days... But we can't survive without breathing for more than a few minutes.

We can't exist without it... But we are never taught how to *use* it!

When prompted, most people think, *"Why would I need to learn about breathing? I know how to breathe, I've done it since the day I was born!"* But most of us really don't know how to breathe *well* and we hold on to unhealthy breathing patterns for our entire lives. The majority of us use less than a third of our lung capacity most of the time.

Like diet, exercise and sleep, breathing is a natural, essential part of being human. And just like these other elements, it can be enhanced with practice and discipline for huge benefits.

We take around 20,000 breaths a day. That's 20,000 opportunities to take control of our bodies and minds and live a calmer, more conscious life.

Eastern esoteric traditions like yoga and Chinese medicine have long understood the power of conscious breathing.

Modern science is not only proving the miraculous health claims of the yogis to be true – it is adding to the story with astounding new studies.

We are only just uncovering the true benefits and techniques of breathwork and we will explore some of the latest research findings in this book.

The exercises in *Draw Breath* are designed to deepen the connection between your body, mind and breath. With the help of fun, relaxing creative challenges, we will explore and unlock the techniques that allow us to master our brains and bodies using our breath.

It's not an airway... ... it's a pathway

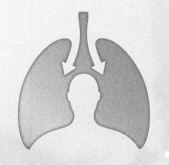

The breath is the only part of your body's autonomic nervous system that can be consciously controlled. But through conscious breathing, you can influence, regulate and balance all of the others. It's a doorway into the parts of yourself you feel you have no control over, **a secret pathway into the subconscious, hidden in plain sight.**

Body–Mind **connection**

UNHAPPY FACES ARE GENERALLY FROWNED UPON

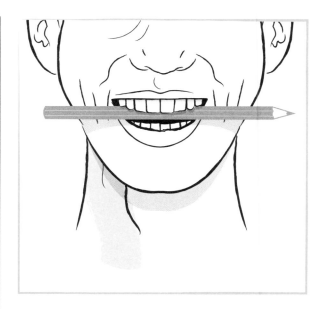

Hold your pencil sideways in your mouth so that it rests past your incisors, between your second or third molars.

Gently bite down with just enough pressure to hold it in place.

You should feel some light tension as the pencil stretches the corners of your mouth, but there shouldn't be any pain or discomfort. If there is, place the pencil further forward in your mouth.

Leaving your pencil in place, take five relaxed breaths, in and out, through your nose.

Noticed any effects?

As well as having aching cheeks, people often find they are smiling after this exercise. Not only that, but they actually report *feeling* happier! In coercing your face into a smile, you have created a positive emotional state.

The body has changed the mind!

If just a few muscles in your cheeks can have this effect, imagine the impact the posture of your entire body is having on your internal state.

Note: I'm not suggesting you should walk around all day with a pencil in your mouth or fake a smile in the hope that it makes you happy (although you are welcome to try!). This exercise is here to illustrate the almost invisible power the body has over the mind.

Mind–Body connection

FOOD FOR THOUGHT

What's your favourite food?

Is there a special dish from your local takeaway that you eat every week? Perhaps it's a home-cooked meal a loved one makes for you. Or do you reward yourself with fine cuisine at a local restaurant as a treat? Is it Indian? Or Italian? Spicy, or sugary sweet?

If you could eat anything right now, in this moment, what would it be?

Take a few minutes to describe, in detail, the vibrant colours, mouth-watering smells and wonderful flavours of your go-to indulgence. Jot down your description on the plate opposite.

Write as though you have been asked to create the menu for a fancy restaurant.

It will help you a great deal if you close your eyes and picture the dish vividly in your mind's eye. Imagine taking a deep breath, inhaling its imaginary aromas through your nose, before loading up your imaginary fork and enjoying an imaginary mouthful.

If you have time, you can even write about dessert!

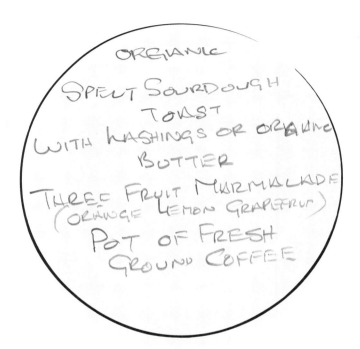

Did you notice any changes in your body as you pictured the food and wrote?

Did you begin to salivate as though the food was in front of you? Did you feel hungrier than you did before? Some people even report their stomach rumbling as they picture their favourite food. None of these responses are likely to shock you, but isn't it interesting that all of these *real*, physical effects were caused by an object that exists only in the mind? This is the power of the mind over the body... Imagine what other effects your imagination is having on your reality!

13

A CRACKPOT IDEA

Before we begin the drawing and breathing exercises, I'd like to say a few things about perfection.

In the Western world we often confuse the concepts of modernity with those of beauty.

We expect everything to be smooth and precise, planned and symmetrical. Not just in our aesthetics but in our lives and our bodies as well. We can feel disappointed when things do not echo these qualities.

Traditional Zen Buddhism teaches us to reflect on the instinctive cycles and spontaneous patterns in nature as meditations on our own impermanence and the organic beauty of the imperfect.

Nature has an inherent capacity for balance and cyclical renewal without the need for symmetry, perpetuity or perfection.

Mistakes are natural. Something to be noticed and learned from so we can grow. They give life its texture. How boring life would be if everything went smoothly all the time!

If at any point in this book your drawing looks absolutely perfect, the chances are, you're doing it wrong. Every breath is unique. Every movement reflects your being as another organic part of nature's pattern. This quality should be revealed as you translate your experience to the page.

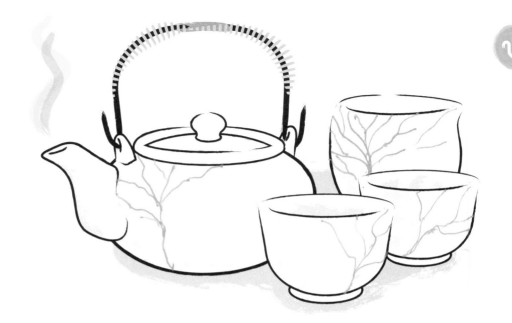

In Japan, this Zen tradition evolved into the concept of "wabi sabi"; the aesthetic appreciation of the imperfect and the impermanent, an alien notion that is not easily translated into our culture of perfectionism.

The Japanese have a tradition in which broken ceramics are repaired with gold, highlighting their imperfections and vulnerabilities rather than attempting to make them invisible. Decorated by the natural, organic beauty of the spontaneous shatter pattern, the reconstructed vessel becomes more beautiful than the original. This art is called "kintsugi" and embodies the aesthetic principles of wabi sabi by teaching us to gild our flaws rather than hide them.

With a yellow or ochre pencil, or a metallic gold pen if you have one, etch some deliberate cracks into this tea set.

Look at the branches of a tree for inspiration for the shapes of the cracks. Notice how similar the organic shapes a tree makes are to those of a fractured ceramic.

If there are no trees in sight, use the patterns of the natural lines in the palm of your hand.

You can even look away from the page as you draw if you'd like the lines to be truly serendipitous.

LISTEN CAREFULLY

Place the tip of your pencil on the dot in the centre of the page.

Close your eyes and take a few moments to listen to the sound of your own breathing.

After three breaths, begin to move the pencil up and down the page in natural flowing movements in time with the breath.

Keeping your eyes closed, see if you can match the sound of the graphite moving across the paper to the sound of the air going in and out through your nose.

Continue this for ten breath cycles, or more if you wish. Remember, don't worry about the image you're creating, this is all about noticing and matching the sound of your breath.

You may find that loosening your grip on the pencil allows your movements to become smoother and quieter.

What can you tell about your internal state from the sound of your breathing?

Throughout this book we will be viewing the pencil as an extension of the breath. As though the movement of your wrist is animated and controlled by your breathing.

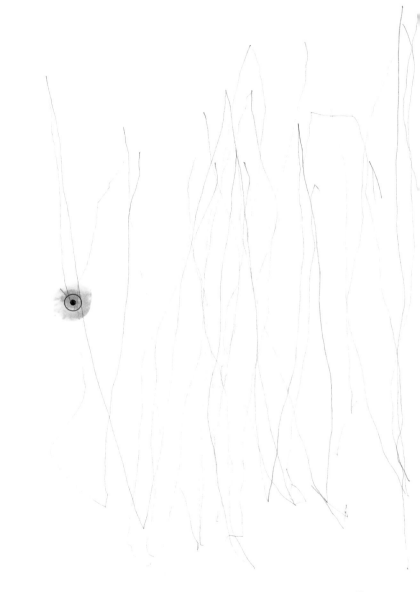

The method

An introduction to drawing breath

In its rawest form, art is a tool for human beings to interpret and express their experience of the world. The simple techniques taught in *Draw Breath* are used to interpret and express the most direct of our experiences – our inner world.

The methods in this book are used for noticing and recording our experience of the breath, with curiosity and compassion, in each moment, as it unfolds.

These simple instructions are key to getting the most out of *Draw Breath*. There will be short reminders throughout the book, but I recommend coming back and reading this page again later on.

The breath should always lead the pencil... never the other way around.

This technique is fundamental to every page in *Draw Breath*. It's the reason I ask you not to jump ahead to the more advanced practices until you have practised a few of the simpler exercises.

When drawing, aim to represent your breathing pattern as though you are observing a model or a landscape and drawing from life. The breath is our subject and requires close and honest observation. **The speed of your breathing should always determine the speed of your drawing.** These exercises should never feel rushed.

If at any point you find yourself speeding up your breathing to complete a practice more quickly, stop. Come back to it later when you have more time.

Before each exercise

Take your time when reading the instructions for each practice and ensure that you understand the key elements.

Before you begin an exercise, pick up your pencil and position the pencil nib on the starting dot on the page. Then, without moving it, take three slow breaths, in and out, paying close attention to the sensation of your breathing. After observing these three breath cycles, begin to move your pencil.

This part of the process is like watching an escalator before you get on it; you are preparing to match your movements to its speed. While some exercises will help you to create a rhythm in your breath, you are *always* aiming to match your drawing speed to the speed of your breath.

Once you have practised this a few times, you can use this calming prelude to check in with your body, check out how you're feeling and notice your state of mind, wherever you are.

After each exercise

Before removing your pencil from the page, take your time to observe at least one breath cycle. Notice how you are feeling after each practice; do you feel any different to before you started? Take note of your mind. How busy is it? What thoughts are there? And your body? What emotions are you feeling? Where are you feeling them? Take as many breaths as feels necessary with this step.

These before and after elements may be difficult to remember but you may find they can become the most informative and rewarding moments. I have included reminders throughout the book.

Introducing the four kinds of exercises...

1. GUIDED

During guided exercises you will be prompted to move your pencil up along the pink dotted line on your inhalation and down the blue dotted line on your exhalation.

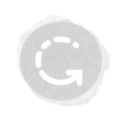

These activities are designed to support a natural flowing rhythm to your breath, to allow you to study its natural pace and to make the internal feedback of the breath easy to notice, one moment at a time.

Guided practices will help you to explore different elements of breath anatomy, psychology and philosophy, and offer focused, relaxing and rhythmic breathing experiences.

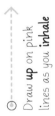
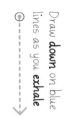

Draw up on pink lines as you inhale

Draw down on blue lines as you exhale

2. FREE-BREATHING

Free-breathing exercises ask you to study your own breath and create a visual account of it using the patterns and breathing techniques you have learned in the guided practices.

The goal here is to allow your drawing to be a true representation of your breath on the page. The more imperfect the drawing, the more accurate it is likely to be as a reflection of the organic fluctuations in your body.

Often, a free-breathing exercise will prompt you to complete an existing illustration by drawing an honest account of your own breath.

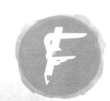

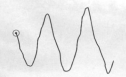

Draw up as you inhale and down as you exhale

3. BREATH-DRAWING

Indicated by solid blue and pink lines. These require a lot of concentration and are more challenging than they seem at first glance. Unlike most guided practices, the blue and pink lines can vary widely in length.

The aim of these activities is to match the speed of your pencil to the rhythm of your breath – no matter the length of the line.

Observe the natural rate of breathing without changing it, while simultaneously varying the speed of your pencil as you trace the image. It can feel a bit like trying to pat your head and rub your belly at the same time to begin with!

If you find these exercises are making your breathing uneven, you are allowing your drawing speed to control the breath and not the other way around. These exercises are best attempted after you are comfortable with the first two types.

The starting dot indicates whether to begin on an inhalation or an exhalation

4. UNIQUE

These one-off activities are spread throughout the book and are accompanied by a specific stated purpose.

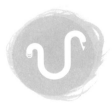

Some unique exercises do not involve the breath at all and instead help you to explore your awareness or your focus, or help to illustrate an abstract point in an experiential way. Pay close attention to the instructions on the unique exercises to get the most out of them.

Getting the most out of *Draw Breath*

Start at the beginning

Draw Breath is ideally completed from front to back. Each task builds on those that have come before it, with the aim of gradually increasing your confidence and understanding.

It's especially recommended that you carry out the first section of the book before completing the rest. It will teach you the basic techniques and help you to become comfortable with the exercises that come later in the book. It will also help you to understand the physiology of your own breathing and build a foundation for some of the information that comes later in the book.

Understanding the basics will help you to get a lot more out of the later practices. Once you're comfortably "drawing breath", feel free to jump ahead to any breath-drawing exercises that call out to you!

Take your time and read the instructions for each individual practice... Every exercise is subtly different.

Share your creations
#DrawBreathBook

When to use *Draw Breath*

In an age of abundance, the one resource we never seem to have enough of is time. Whether we are replying to a never-ending barrage of emails, chauffeuring kids around or squeezing in a quick grocery dash, finding even ten minutes to ourselves can seem impossible. The very idea of trying to find time can make us feel stressed. However, if you do these exercises, and find them relaxing, they will create their own time. When you feel relaxed you are more productive and you will find that your time is easier to manage.

Many of the exercises in this book will take under a minute to complete, while others are designed so that you can come back and continue to build on your drawing as many times as you like.

In terms of what time of day is appropriate, it goes without saying that your body has its own natural rhythms. Breathing exercises that balance the nervous system tend to help the body to carry out whatever important tasks it's naturally engaged in; whether problem solving or preparing for sleep, balancing the mind and body will help you perform better. Practising these tasks in the morning may help you to de-stress and feel more focused for whatever you may be facing that day. Meanwhile, practising in the evening may feel restorative and prepare your mind and body for rest. See what works for you.

What drawing tool to use

Although I use the word "pencil" throughout the book, I encourage you to try as many different drawing tools as you like. Explore the different expectations, sensations and results that come with using each one, and find what feels right for you.

Personally, I prefer using a humble pencil (or its futuristic cousin the mechanical pencil) for free-breathing exercises. A pencil is inherently tactile and will give you tangible feedback from the texture of the page, with the added benefit that you can rub it out and repeat the task if you like! Ink pens can be more rewarding for guided practices, allowing you to create smooth, fluid motions across the page.

I leave colours entirely up to you and hope that selecting different hues depending on the task will add a fun creative element to help make the exercises your own. Experiment!

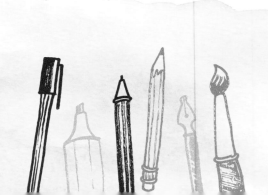

How to use *Draw Breath*

Sit in an upright and alert posture at a raised table. Keep your chin tucked in to lengthen the back of your neck, but do not face your head down toward the book in a way that arches your spine. Aim to keep your shoulders relaxed throughout.

This book is designed as a hardback so that it can be used anywhere. I suggest you aim to create a peaceful environment, free from distractions, where you are unlikely to be disturbed by family members, pets or your smartphone.

Sitting on the ground with crossed legs in a traditional meditation position is only recommended if it is comfortable for your body to sit like this for more than a short period of time. If you do wish to sit in a cross-legged or lotus position, place the book on a raised area in front of you to avoid arching your back to reach the page.

There are many ways of using this book, and what works for one person may not work for another. It may help to raise the book by placing it on top of other books. The key is finding a position in which you feel comfortable, alert and calm, where your shoulders are relaxed and your breathing is unhindered by a slouching posture.

Keep your posture upright and alert to maximize space in your lungs and allow for deep diaphragmatic breathing.

Audio content

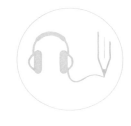

All of the practices within *Draw Breath* can be completed by following the simple instructions. However, audio support is available for free at drawbreath.com for the paced exercises, such as coherent breathing, and some of the guided meditation practices. Similar to traditional guided meditations, these recordings are helpful when you'd like to really take your time and pace your breathing accurately. Where a task has the option for audio support you will see the headphones symbol shown above.

A patchwork of practices

Draw Breath is unashamedly eclectic in nature. I have scoured different traditions, scientific and spiritual, ancient and new, from around the world, selecting interesting insights and inspirations and reinterpreting them through the lens of illustration, in an attempt to bring you a rich and diverse introduction to different breathing methods, meditations and philosophies.

I hope that this approach demonstrates two things. Firstly (despite many claims to the contrary), no *one* tradition "owns" breathing as a method of meditation or relaxation. Secondly, due to our common physiology, breathing exercises have universal appeal and utility across cultures and time. A twelfth-century Sufi mystic, a modern Japanese student or a Western businesswoman will undergo the same predictable, physical and, likely, emotional changes when engaging in a breathing practice. The breath is not just a means of unifying the body and mind, it is a unifying force between human beings.

The benefits of breathwork
a quick summary

"Breathwork" refers to the deliberate control of your breathing pattern or simply the conscious awareness of your breath in its natural state.

Conscious breathing can improve your focus, help you to relax and increase your energy levels.

These each have wider benefits, from the physical to the mental, and eventually, even the spiritual.

If there was a magic pill that had all of these incredible benefits, with no negative side effects, how much would you be willing to pay for it?

The good news is, you don't have to. Air is free and all around you. The breath is always available to you, and always will be.

On a **physical** level it can...

- Relax your body
- Improve your sleep
- Increase your energy levels
- Relieve muscle tension
- Increase your stamina
- Reduce inflammation
- Improve blood pressure
- Reduce the risk of heart attacks and strokes
- Naturally remove toxins from your body through the lungs
- Reduce and even subtly reverse the effects of aging (see p68!)
- Strengthen and stretch your muscles, improving posture and protecting you from back, knee and hip injuries
- Be used to release and let go of suppressed emotions and past traumas stored in the body as tension

On a **mental** level it can...

- Clear your mind
- Increase positive thoughts
- Improve positive emotions
- Help you to recognize and break negative thought patterns
- Create feelings of inner peace
- Help you to feel calm and balanced
- Increase resilience and self-esteem
- Improve internal sensory capabilities and self-awareness
- Deepen intuition
- Increase your capacity for creative insights
- Make you feel more connected to the people around you
- Make you more present to deal with life's problems and enjoy its riches

How does it work?

This list of benefits might sound unbelievable, but the more you think about it, the more it starts to make sense.

Increasing the oxygen levels in your bloodstream keeps your cells healthy and supports tissue growth in your organs and muscles.

The movement of healthy breathing engages your muscles, massages your vital organs and circulates the lymphatic system while cleansing the bloodstream by releasing CO_2 and other toxins through the lungs.

Deep breathing relaxes, strengthens and stretches muscles that subtly affect posture. Healthy breathing requires good posture and good posture requires healthy breathing. The two are complementary counterparts. Posture and breath both reflect and affect your mood and blood chemistry.

Slow, rhythmic breathing activates the parasympathetic nervous system (PNS).

The PNS controls most of the systems that keep your internal organs in balance with each other – your *homeostasis*. It also "switches off" your fight-or-flight response, which allows your body to enter "rest-and-digest" mode, strengthening all of your natural homeostatic functions even further, from your blood pressure to your immune system. It even improves how effectively you absorb the nutrients from your food.

The more effectively and rhythmically you breathe, the stronger these benefits will be for your body and mind.

Breathwork isn't just about removing the negative, it is an instrument for balancing our internal physical and mental states and taking us above and beyond our expectations of ourselves to live our best possible lives.

The breath can heal us and improve our well-being physically, emotionally and spiritually. This book introduces the "how" and the "why" gradually, through fun, creative and intrinsically relaxing exercises.

Breathing... the basics

What are the variables of the breath that we can notice and control?

There are many different qualities to the breath, each with its own subtle effect on the body and mind. As you read each of the following factors, take a few moments to check in and notice how each one manifests in your breath in this moment.

Rate

How fast do you breathe? How frequent are your breaths? This is often measured in "breaths per minute". The slower you breathe, the fewer breaths per minute you take. In healthy people, breathing slowly is a sign of relaxed contentment.

Depth

Is your breathing deep or shallow? How much air are you actually taking in? In scientific literature this is called "tidal volume". When combined with the rate and ratio, alterations to depth can have a huge impact on our focus and energy levels.

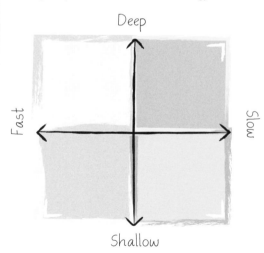

How does your breathing look at the moment?
Is it deep or shallow? Fast or slow?
Check in with yourself and mark an X on the chart.

Ratio

Which is longer? Your inhale? Or your exhale? At usual resting rate our out-breath is often marginally longer than our in-breath. This ratio can be consciously controlled for different effects on the body and nervous system. Longer inhalations are dynamic and energizing, while longer exhalations are relaxing and restorative.

Count the seconds for your next inhalation and exhalation. Which is longer?

Rhythm

How regular is your breathing? Are you breathing in strong rhythmic cycles? Or do you take a few breaths and then hold for a while, perhaps while concentrating, before gasping in or sighing out your next breath? As we will see later in the book, deliberate, rhythmic breathing has astounding health benefits, while unconscious sighing may be a sign of overexertion.

Pauses

Do you notice a short pause after your exhalation? If so, how long is the pause? How does it feel to extend it? Does it feel more relaxing? Or uncomfortable? How does it feel to briefly hold the air in your lungs after you inhale?

Texture

Is the gentle movement of your body smooth as you inhale and exhale? Or is it uneven and stuttering? When we are upset our breath can become very erratic, especially when we cry. The smoother the breath, the more relaxed the body and mind.

Location

Do you breathe into your lower abdomen? Or your upper chest? Do your shoulders and ribcage move when you breathe? Or does your belly expand? What muscles are you using to do this? Are you tensing your muscles? Or relaxing them?

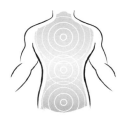

What location on your body are you breathing "into"?

Circle the "centre" of your breath on this image.

Quality

Is your breathing laboured or painful? Does it require effort or exertion? Or is it breezy and easy? Sometimes we use effort on the exhale, sometimes it is a simple matter of relaxing. Sometimes we feel short of breath and the more effort we try to make, the more difficult breathing seems to become.

Oral vs nasal

Do you naturally breathe through your mouth or your nose? Neither is "wrong", but nasal breathing is considered more conducive to health. Each breath's path can be selected or combined for different effects. For example, breathing in through the nose to filter and warm the air, then exhaling smoothly through the mouth with pursed lips to create soothing resistance.

Nostril dominance

Your nostrils take turns to subtly expand and contract in a cycle that lasts around one hour. When dominant, each nostril strengthens and supports activity in the opposite brain hemisphere. For example, when the left nostril is dominant, the right side of your brain is more active, and you are subtly more emotionally attuned and better at lateral thinking.[1]

Automatic vs deliberate

Do you have to think about breathing in? Are you breathing consciously or unconsciously now? Has the question shifted you from automatic to deliberate breathing? Neither of these is "correct". This book will explore both conscious, deliberate breathing exercises and prompts that ask you to "watch" your body's natural, automatic breathing cycle.

Throughout the book I refer to "breath cycles". A breath cycle includes one inhalation and one exhalation.

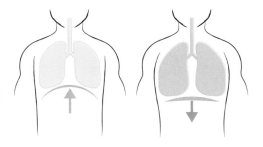

As we breathe in, the diaphragm draws down and our ribs expand, creating a vacuum that pulls air into our lungs. We can also use our chest, back and shoulder muscles to breathe: this is so that we can take short, fast breaths when we are in danger or need to move quickly.

We can become aware of all of these factors and each can be consciously altered to create a different desired effect.

Throughout *Draw Breath* you will explore the various ways controlling and observing your breath affects your body and mind.

"Type" of breath

Gasp? Yawn? Sigh? These (often involuntary) breathing styles have their own unique evolutionary purposes that we will discuss later on. Sobbing with tears or doubling over with laughter are essentially *styles of breathing*. They are evidence of how fundamentally connected our emotions are to our breath... and our bodies to our minds.

Airway resistance

Do you have a blocked nose or sore throat? Notice how this affects your breathing and energy levels... right when you need your energy the most!

On a less temporary scale, muscle tension and tightness in our backs and abdominal muscles can also impact on the depth and location of our breathing. Slowly, over time, with the right techniques, the act of breathing itself can reduce this tightness, creating space in the body and expanding our lung capacity.

What does healthy breathing look like?

Often, in stressful situations, someone with good intentions will prompt us to take a deep breath.

When someone tells you to take a deep breath, what do you do? Go ahead... Take a deep breath...

Most of us, when told to take a deep breath, hastily suck in our bellies, taking a short, fast, audible breath, in through the mouth, puffing up the chest, raising our shoulders and using the muscles in the back and upper chest... In other words... the exact opposite of a relaxing breath.

In fact, this type of breathing is an exaggerated version of what the body naturally does when we are feeling stressed or anxious.

When we are relaxed, our breathing shows the polar opposite behaviour – we breathe slowly, using the diaphragm to draw air in through the nose and down toward the belly, in long, smooth, rhythmic breaths. This is the kind of breathing we should aim for when we are told to "take a deep breath". It may help to think more about taking a *slow* breath, than a *deep* one.

Stressed breathing

- Fast, short breaths
- Oral
- More audible / harsh sounding
- Breathing into the upper chest using the upper back and intercostal muscles
- The breath becomes choppy and uneven.
- Alternatively, the breath freezes completely, followed by gasps/sighs

Relaxed breathing

- Long, slow breaths
- Nasal
- Soft, smooth sounds
- Breathing into the belly using the diaphragm
- Regular, even, rhythmic cycles

Bad breath causes injury...

When we don't use our full breathing capacity on a regular basis, our natural breathing muscles not only become weaker, they become tighter because they are not being stretched through their full range of motion. This forces the body to rely on the smaller, more easily fatigued intercostal and shoulder muscles to breathe, causing tension, back injuries and chronic pain. All of our muscles are connected; when the diaphragm becomes tight, the psoas muscle, which connects the diaphragm to the hips and pelvis, can tighten too, leading to hip and knee problems.

Breathing health is integral to safe posture.

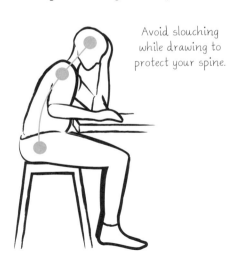

Avoid slouching while drawing to protect your spine.

Breathing into the upper chest is an adaptive evolutionary response to threat. It helps the body prepare to hyperventilate for fast movement, or freeze and play dead as the fight-or-flight response kicks in. The hallmarks of stressed breathing can be positive in small doses, making us more alert and giving us a burst of energy. This is great for focusing during problem solving or for boosting our performance when we're playing sports.

In the evolutionary environment of our ancestors, this state of breathing would have only been active for a few minutes, or, in extreme circumstances, hours, until the threat had passed and their internal physiology returned to rest-and-digest mode.

But in our chronically stressed modern world where we can perceive abstract things like deadlines, bills and job security as subtle but ever-present threats, we are able to sustain elements of these intense or frozen breathing styles for hours, days or even years. The breathing pattern itself sends signals back up to the brain telling it that we are under threat, causing further anxiety and creating a negative cycle that we are often unaware that we are in!

It's not just stress that causes this pattern of unhealthy breathing. Sitting for long hours at a desk, driving a car, or watching TV are all unnatural positions for the body to be in for extended periods of time. Slumping your head and shoulders forward and bending your spine pushes your belly down and reduces your body's natural breathing space, forcing you to breathe higher up in your ribcage.

Breathwork exercises help you to become more aware of your breath in daily life, allowing you to notice bad patterns and replace them with healthy ones.

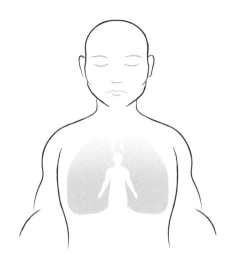

What does all of this say about you?

Who ever thought that breathing could sound so complicated!

All of these distinct aspects of your breathing combine to create your unique moment-to-moment breath quality. They are outward indicators of your internal state – you can tell a lot about your emotional state and energy levels by simply observing the elements of your breath.

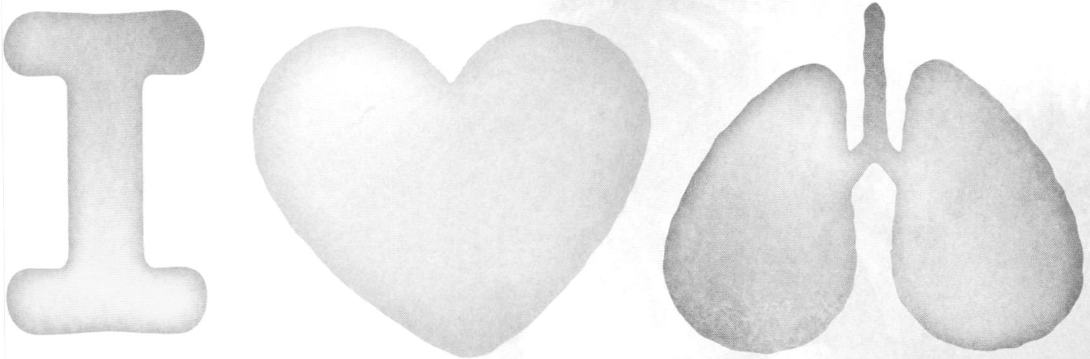

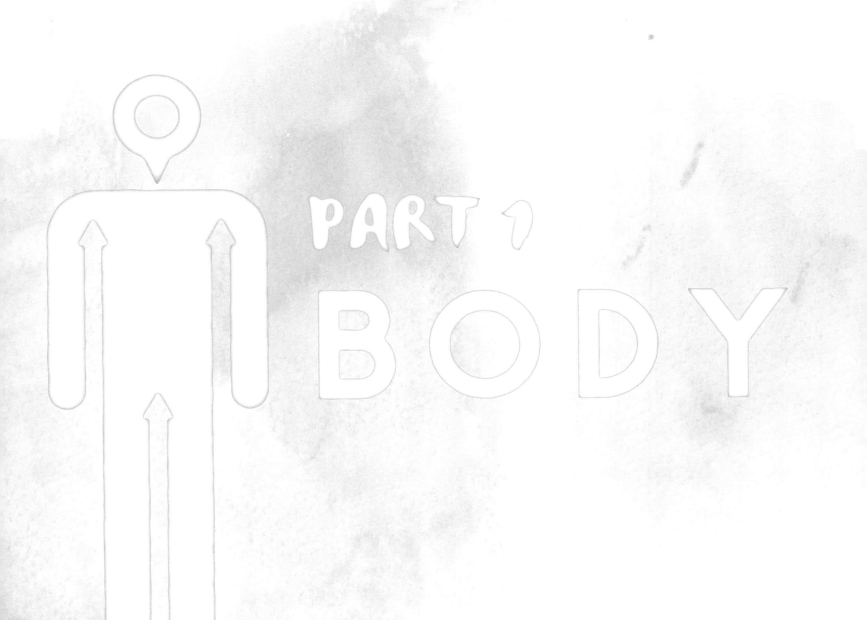

PART 1

BODY

"Much of the secret
of life consists in
knowing how to
laugh, and also
how to breathe."

– Alan Watts

WHERE DO YOU BREATHE?

Place one hand on your belly and the other on your heart. Observe a few breaths in your natural breathing pattern. Which moves more? The hand on your belly, or the hand on your heart? Or do only your shoulders move? In the West, by the time most of us are adults we have developed the unhealthy habit of breathing exclusively into our chests.

For this exercise, place the tip of your pencil on the page in the starting dot.

Next, place the book in your lap, and position the other end of your pencil on your belly, about halfway between your sternum and your belly button. Now breathe out fully.

Now breathe in with the intention of pushing your pencil as far as you can up the page with your inflating belly, drawing a straight line with the movement.

If it is moving across the paper even a little bit, you are successfully breathing into your belly.

Repeat in a different colour, this time more slowly. Instead of aiming to force your belly out, intentionally relax your abdominal muscles and pull down your diaphragm... Did the pencil move further?

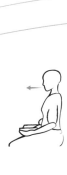

Hold the bottom of the page against your belly and place the tip of your pencil on the starting point.

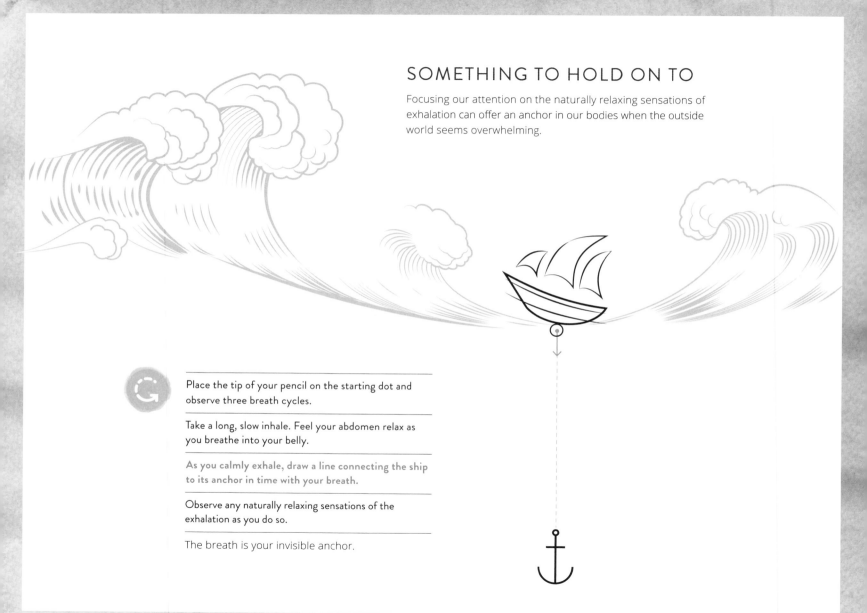

SOMETHING TO HOLD ON TO

Focusing our attention on the naturally relaxing sensations of exhalation can offer an anchor in our bodies when the outside world seems overwhelming.

Place the tip of your pencil on the starting dot and observe three breath cycles.

Take a long, slow inhale. Feel your abdomen relax as you breathe into your belly.

As you calmly exhale, draw a line connecting the ship to its anchor in time with your breath.

Observe any naturally relaxing sensations of the exhalation as you do so.

The breath is your invisible anchor.

STAY GROUNDED

When we contemplate the beauty of a lotus flower floating on the surface of a lake, we often fail to consider its stem. The shoot of the lotus is always there, below the surface, providing it with nutrients and grounding it into the earth.

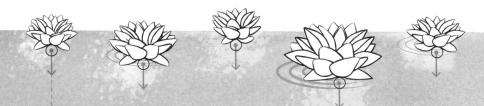

Connect these lotus flowers to the bed of the lake.

Draw a line from the starting circle on the first flower to the circle below it. Repeat for each flower over five successive exhalations.

Match the speed of your pencil to your exhalation as it unfolds. Take as long to draw the line as it takes to exhale.

Search your body for the naturally relaxing sensations of the breath, feel your limbs grow heavier as you exhale. Allow this heaviness to ground you wherever your body is in contact with the floor or chair.

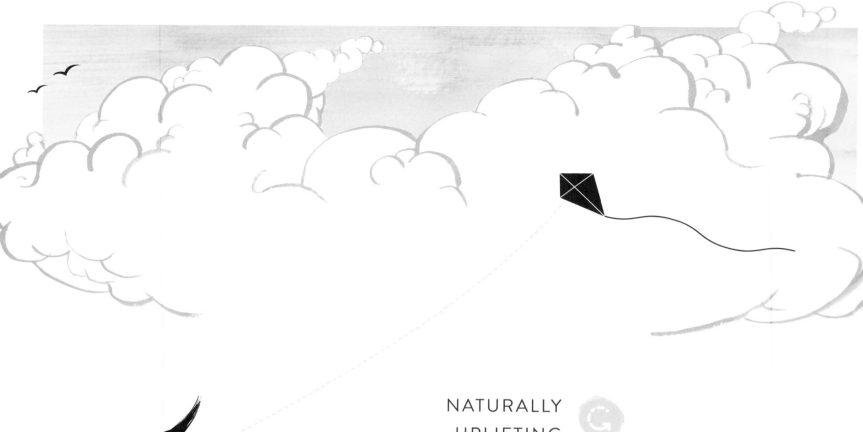

NATURALLY
UPLIFTING

Inhaling oxygen invigorates and energizes us.
Breathing deep into the belly naturally lifts
our posture and with it our mood.

Breathe out smoothly. Notice the
natural pause at the end of your
exhalation.

Upon inhaling, slowly connect this
girl's line to her kite as it floats.

Feel your body expand and lift from your
belly to your upper chest as you do so.

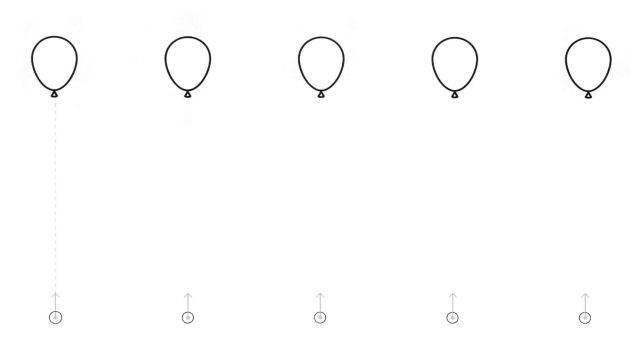

RISE WITH THE IN-BREATH

For five successive inhalations, draw a line from the starting circle to the balloon. Feel how your torso naturally lifts and expands, and notice your spine lengthen as you breathe in.

Take as long to draw the line as it takes to inhale, as though the movement of your breath in your belly is moving the pencil across the page.

To explore further, visualize a string with a balloon attached coming out from the crown of your head. Imagine it gently lifting you through the centre line of your body as you inhale.

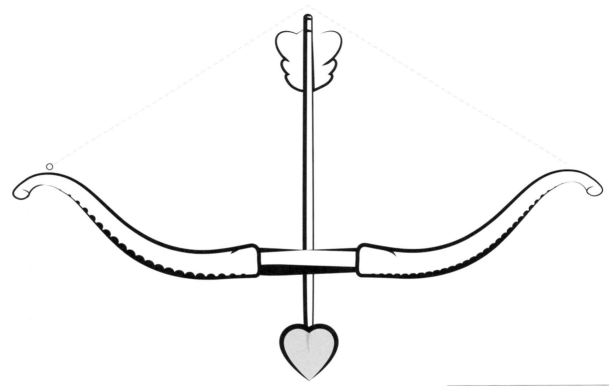

DRAW BACK YOUR BOW

As you breathe in, the diaphragm activates, pulling down and creating a vacuum in your lungs that pulls air in through the airway. As you breathe out, the diaphragm relaxes and releases, moving back into its starting position, pushing the air out.

As you draw the upstroke of this bowstring, feel your diaphragm drawing down and creating space in your lungs as you inhale.

When you reach the top, relax and "let go" of the diaphragm and observe how effortlessly your body exhales, letting go of the tension you have created as you complete the downstroke.

An active inhalation allows for a passive and relaxed exhalation.

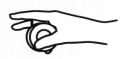

MOMENTUM

When aiming to take a "deep" breath, rather than attempting to inhale forcefully, we can use the organic momentum of the exhalation to instigate a naturally long and deep inhalation.

If we take one conscious exhalation, breathing out *fully* and noticing the natural pause at the end of the exhalation, then wait for the body's own urge to inhale, our breathing naturally deepens and lengthens.

As you exhale fully, draw the string connecting the hand to the yo-yo.

Take your time and pause momentarily once the line connects to the yo-yo. "Send" the yo-yo back up on your inhalation, noticing any effects that the long, deep exhalation has had on this fresh inhalation.

Repeat this process for a few more breaths, tracing over your original lines, noticing the effect that the length of each breath has on the next.

Without speeding up your breathing, combine the techniques on this spread to see if you can create momentum with your breath.

Allow your inhalation to be passive in the beginning and then inhale fully with effort... Begin a passive exhale, then exhale fully with effort...

In other words, only actively breathe at the very end of your inhalations and exhalations. The vacuum left by the exhalation causes the next inhalation and the force of the volume of air in the lungs starts the exhalation.

See how little effort you can use to breath fully in this way.

Notice the expansive, uplifting sensations of your next in-breath and the grounding, relaxing sensations of your next out-breath.

LEARNING CURVES

Place the tip of your pencil at base of the arc and breathe out.

Breathe in and follow the arc with your pencil as though you're indicating the fill level of your lungs until you reach the peak.

When you reach the peak, pause momentarily and let your exhalation guide your pencil down the arc.

The dotted lines are only guides. The more you stray, the truer you are being to your breath.

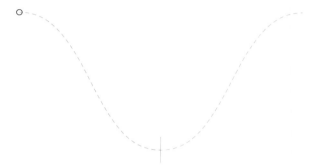

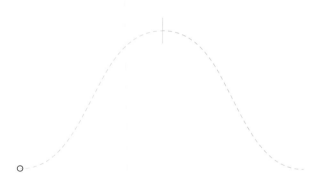

Remember to observe three natural breath cycles before moving your pencil.

BETTER OUT THAN IN?

We often perceive our breath as beginning on an inhalation, but it makes just as much sense to experience the exhalation as the start. The breath is a constant flow, not a single unit.

Repeat the previous illustration, but this time begin on an exhalation.

Do you notice any differences when perceiving the breath this way?

There is a natural pause as you complete your exhalation. You may wish to stop moving your pencil at this point, or alternatively, draw a flat line to indicate this.

RIDE THE WAVE OF THE BREATH

It may help to imagine the breath as a wave and yourself as a surfer. Sometimes you will lose concentration and roll under, distracted by daydreams as the wave rolls ahead.

You can always get back on the crest by focusing on your breath in this moment.

Put together the exercises we have done so far, linking together one breath after the other in a continuing line.

If you lose concentration, simply "get back on the board".

Take your time on this page. Let your breath set the pace.

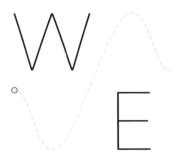

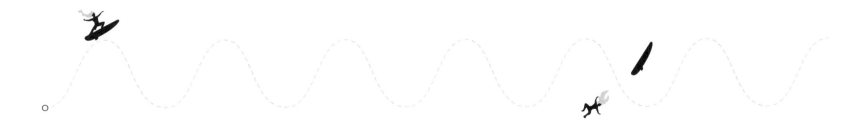

SET YOURSELF FREE

It's time for your first free-breathing exercise!

Just like a seismograph measures the vibrations of the earth, the aim is to let your pencil become a true reflection of the fluctuations in your breath as you move it across the page. The purpose of the exercise is not to create a completely accurate representation. No one is marking your work. The point is to deepen your capacity to focus on every moment of your breath, in real time, as each moment passes into the next.

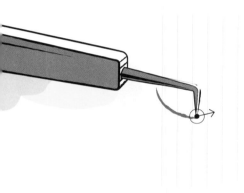

Place the tip of your pencil on the dot at the tip of the seismograph and observe three calm breaths before beginning to move your pencil to the right.

Allow your breath to define its own natural rhythm. You are not trying to control it, you are simply watching it in its automatic state.

Draw up and down to indicate depth, and across to indicate speed. Keep going until you reach the edge of the page.

Notice and record the minute differences in each curve. Every breath is unique.

You may wish to close your eyes and draw an image solely based on *feeling* so that you don't get distracted by the "quality" of your drawing.

Your breath is unlikely to be a perfect arc. And your out-breath may not be equal to your in-breath. Let the arcs reflect the nuances of each breath. The less perfect your curves look, the more likely it is an accurate image of your breath.

Notice your posture as you repeat the practice on this page.

Remember to keep your head raised and your chest open.

You can do this free-breathing exercise anytime, anywhere. All you need is a pencil, a piece of paper and your breath.

Biofeedback

Long before we had wearable technology and pedometers in smartphones, scientists were hooking themselves up to scientific feedback machines and using the data to change their lives.

Biofeedback is a form of therapy developed in the twentieth century in which practitioners receive live audio, visual or touch feedback about an area of their bodies; information about their pulse, their breath, skin conductance or even brain waves.

By observing the live data and comparing it to their subjective experience, practitioners learn to focus on and control or relax the systems and reactions in their own body. For example, one person may sit in front of an ECG that is measuring and giving them a visual representation of their heartbeat. They can use this information to slowly learn how to calm their pulse by focusing on the rate and quality of their breathing.

Biofeedback enhances awareness and control of the mind and body in response to immediate feedback.

Some of the pioneers of biofeedback reference yoga and meditation as the oldest forms of the technique. Of course, yogis rely on their own focus for somatic "data" rather than machines, but the principle is the same: listen to your body and change your focus or behaviour in line with what you're experiencing in real time.

The free-breathing exercises in this book are a form of self-reported biofeedback; a "live" record of the breath is created on the page, training you to be more aware of fluctuations in the breathing experience.

THE BREATH IS A CYCLE

The breath goes around and around... Like a wheel in motion, it appears to propel itself, and us along with it. The inhalation could not exist without the exhalation. They are two halves of a whole, the yin and yang, equalizing each other and creating movement and energy as a result.

Complete as many slow breath cycles as you like while tracing these wheels.

Observe the breath's natural capacity to animate itself without your input. It has its own energy, will and momentum.

Always observe three natural breath cycles without drawing before moving your pencil.

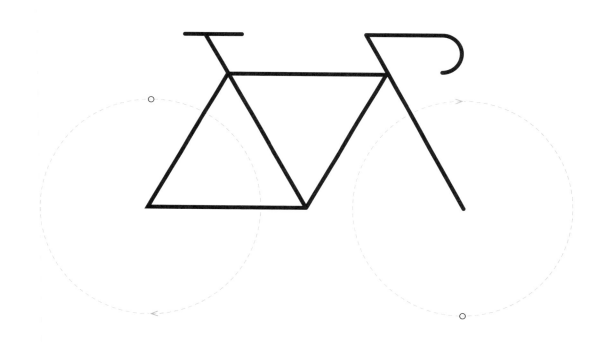

THE MUSIC OF
THE SPHERES

Everything in the universe flows in
musical patterns, from the beating of
your heart and the billowing of your
lungs, to the changing of the seasons
and the clockwork orbiting of the planets
and moons. Nature thrives on rhythm.

Using the circular breath-drawing technique
you have just learned, draw a simple solar
system on this page.

Start with the sun in the centre, then
add concentric circles around it to show
the orbits of the planets. Finally, add
the planets themselves, always using the
rhythm of your own breath as a guide.

Feel free to create your own unique solar
system. You are welcome to include moons
and their orbits too!

ENERGIZING

You may well be going through life unaware that you are not using the full capacity of your lungs.

Even when we know that slow, full breathing is preferable, it can feel unnatural to jump straight from short, shallow breaths to deeper ones.

It can take a few breaths for the necessary muscles to activate and for our body to relax and create space. In these situations, we can take increasingly deep breaths, with each one expanding subtly on the last to ensure a smooth transition.

Connect this cable to its power source using the ebb and flow of your breath.

You may feel your energy levels gradually increasing as you take progressively deeper, calmer breaths. This is because you are oxygenating the blood more thoroughly while remaining at rest.

Breathing in and out in large breaths not only increases your energy but also your focus.

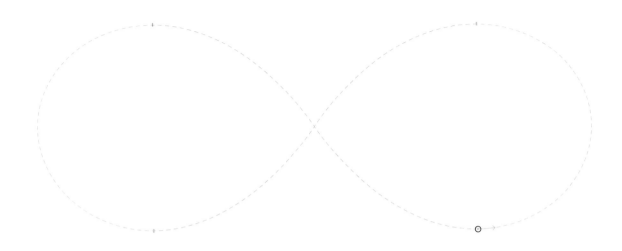

AN INFINITE LOOP

Without thinking or trying, without any conscious effort at all, our breath continues unabated, from our first moments of life to our last.

Starting on an inhalation, begin tracing the bottom right of the loop in time with your breath.

Repeat the pattern as many times as you like.

Once comfortable with the pattern, repeat the symbol on the blank areas of the page as a free-breathing doodle practice.

Does your breath become slower and more rhythmic the more you become aware of it?

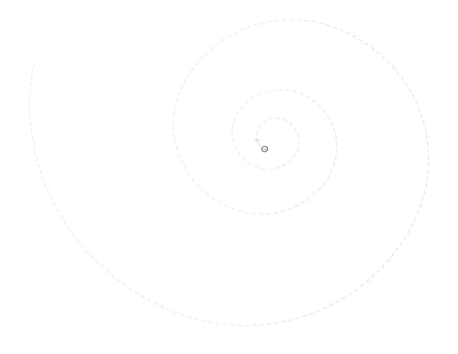

LOWER RATE, HIGHER STATE

Slowing your breathing rate naturally calms your body and mind.

Starting at the centre of the spiral on an inhalation, allow your inhalations and exhalations to become longer and deeper with each loop.

It may help you to slow down your breathing rate if you inhale and exhale fully in each breath cycle.

Does your breath become naturally deeper as you slow down its rate? Once you have completed the spiral, close your eyes and continue breathing with the rhythm and momentum you have built for a few moments.

NATURALLY EXPANDING

The more we begin to tune in to our breath and how it feels, the more peaceful, deeper, longer and healthier it naturally becomes.

Create your own spiral patterns on the page opposite using your breath as a guide.

Think of your spirals as tiny galaxies spinning, growing and expanding.

Experiment with size and direction. You may find that drawing smaller, tighter spirals requires more concentration and naturally slows down your breathing rate.

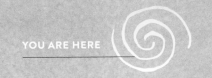

YOU ARE HERE

Two halves of one whole

Fight-or-flight
vs rest-and-digest

Imagine if you had to remember to beat your heart every second, while simultaneously breathing and controlling your digestive system with conscious effort. If your memory and multitasking skills are anything like mine, it wouldn't take long for your body to be fatally out of whack. Luckily, you don't have to do any of these things. Your body takes care of all your essential functions effortlessly.

These bodily processes are controlled by your autonomic nervous system. This network of nerves and neurons runs throughout your body and brain, and, without any conscious input, it regulates and maintains the balance of your internal organs. Put simply, it does all the boring but vital stuff that keeps you alive.

Our essential processes are monitored, channelled and controlled through two distinct but corresponding halves of the autonomic nervous system: the sympathetic nervous system (SNS) and the parasympathetic nervous system (PNS).

The SNS is dynamic and stimulating, while the PNS is calming and relaxing.

The SNS sends signals that "switch on" our muscles, the PNS "switches them off".

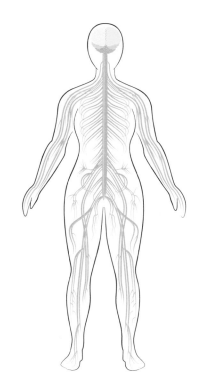

When your mind perceives a threat, whether real or imagined, it sends signals through the SNS that prepare you to stand your ground, or run away quickly. Your heart rate elevates, your breathing rate increases, and blood is directed away from your digestive system toward your large muscles. The chemistry of your body changes as adrenaline and cortisol are released into the bloodstream, preparing you for quick decisive action. In other words, the SNS is responsible for all of the hallmarks of the infamous "fight-or-flight response".

In the industrialized world, our jobs often require us to remain in a constant state of alertness while staying in a sedentary position. This means we never "burn off" the energizing chemicals that we release into the bloodstream in response to stress. Add to this the abstract but ever-present problems our minds perceive as threats – deadlines, job security, complicated home and work schedules – and it's easy to see how, even though we are not visibly in a state of panic, this constant, intense alertness requires the continuous activity of the SNS.

As a result, for many of us, our bodies are in a chronic state of tension.

There is a less famous counterpart to fight-or-flight called the "relaxation response", sometimes referred to as the "rest-and-digest response", which is controlled via the PNS.

When activated, it de-escalates the effects of the SNS. Your heart rate decreases and becomes more rhythmic. Your breath becomes deeper and longer. Blood flows toward your digestive system and internal organs, sharing essential nutrients around the body. When in this state, your body begins to naturally heal itself, focusing on the immune system, controlling inflammation more effectively and releasing its own natural pain killers. Your blood chemistry stabilizes, and you release positive reward hormones such as oxytocin more readily.

So how do we "switch off" the SNS and stimulate the PNS?

The secret power of the breath

The autonomic nervous system is your body's unconscious way of controlling all of the internal patterns that keep it in a state of equilibrium, or "homeostasis". It simultaneously drives:

- The beating of your heart
- Your blood pressure level
- The pattern of your breathing
- The cycle of your hormones
- Your blood chemistry
- The movements of your digestive system
- Your circadian rhythm

You don't have to think about any of these things consciously, yet they are all taken care of...

Have you spotted the odd one out?

Your breath is the only part of this system you have real conscious control over, the only pattern that you can deliberately alter. But by modifying the breath, you can control the other elements of the system. The breath is a doorway into the unconscious systems of the body. By changing your breathing pattern, you can stimulate aspects of both the SNS and PNS, choosing to bring them into balance or activate one more than the other. This affects the entire physiology of your body and its internal systems, as well as the subtle qualities of your mental state, emotional state and the quality of your attention.

Understanding the power of the breath is key to mastery of your physical and mental well-being.

HIJACK YOURSELF!

The breath is a pathway between the body and the mind.

Breathing acts as a control board for the autonomic nervous system, allowing you to send deliberate signals to the brain using specific breathing patterns.

By altering the speed, depth and other qualities of your breathing, you can send a message to your brain that says "everything is OK", which in turn changes your internal physiological state, and with it, your mental state.

This "fake it 'til you make it" strategy interrupts the negative cycles of chronic stress and overrides the SNS response, converting you from a state of fight-or-flight to one of rest-and-digest. You can literally switch your body's internal situation from one of panic to one of calm by "switching on" the PNS with breathwork. When activated, the PNS diverts traffic from the SNS, cancelling out its more acute effects.

As you calmly trace the lung pattern above, imagine the signal travelling from the brain telling the lungs to take two slow, deep breaths, all the way into your diaphragm.

The lungs in turn send a calming signal through the heart and back up to the brain.

What differences do you notice after doing this?

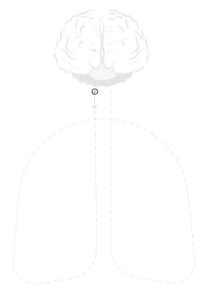

The lowest part of your lungs has the highest number of alveoli, the tiny air sacs where oxygen is absorbed into the bloodstream. So breathing into your belly in a naturally relaxed way helps to fully oxygenate and detoxify the blood.

THREE-PART BREATH

To get the most out of your breath it may be helpful to imagine the space inside your torso is divided into three parts. This is a technique that is often taught in yoga classes.

First, breathe into the bottom of your belly, feeling it naturally expand and make space.

Next, feel your ribcage begin to expand in all directions as it fills with air.

Finally, allow your chest to rise and fill, all the way up to your collarbone.

Control your exhale in reverse order, allowing your chest to drop and release first, and relaxing your diaphragm last of all.

Practise this four times, drawing the path of your breath on the diagrams as though it is the "fill level" of your lungs.

The dots will help you break your breath into thirds.

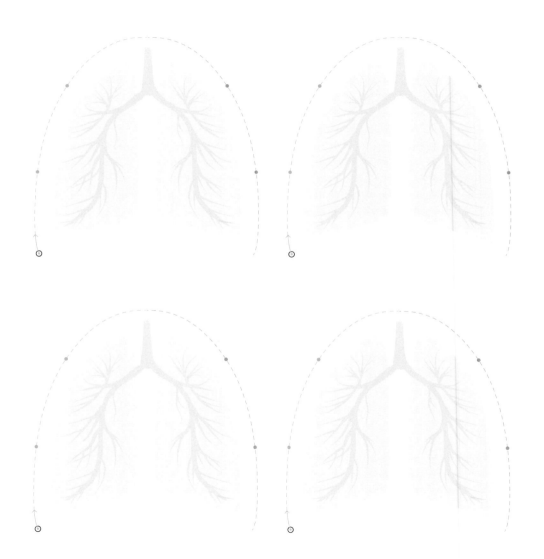

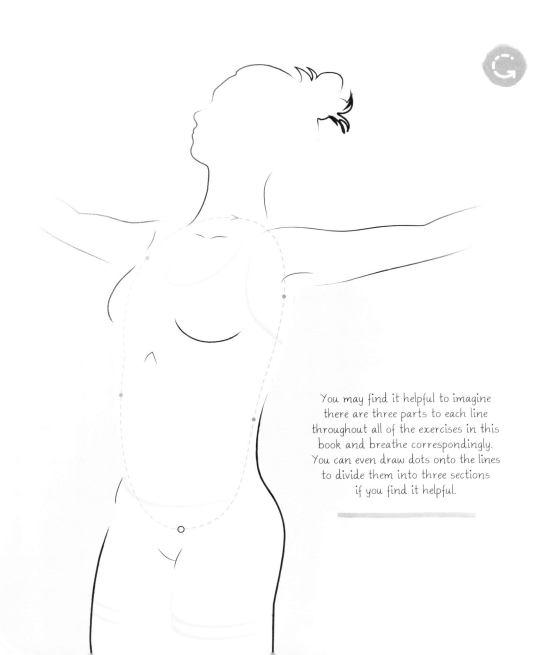

You may find it helpful to imagine there are three parts to each line throughout all of the exercises in this book and breathe correspondingly. You can even draw dots onto the lines to divide them into three sections if you find it helpful.

PRANAYAMA

The breath control and awareness techniques of yoga are called "pranayama" and are considered foundational to yogic practice, even more elemental than the poses, or "asana", that quickly come to mind when picturing a yoga class. The key to mastering asana is to move the body with the rhythm of the breath, expanding each movement and deepening each posture in time with the inhalation and exhalation.

Focus your attention on the muscles of your pelvic floor and feel them subtly relax as you inhale.

Mirror your awareness in your own body with the location of your pencil on the picture as it moves.

As you trace your inhalation, follow the journey of your pencil on the picture up your own abdomen and all the way up your chest, until your lungs are full of air and expanding against your collarbone.

As you exhale, follow the line all the way from your shoulder blades to the base of your spine, feeling each part relax as you trace. Allow your shoulder blades to "melt" down your back as the pencil moves past them.

Finishing where you began, empty your lungs completely and notice the natural engagement of the pelvic floor required to do so.

Slower, deeper breaths transfer more oxygen into the lungs and remove more carbon dioxide, energizing and cleansing the body. We breathe out more than 2 pounds of CO_2 every day!

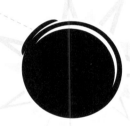

SHORT FUSE?

In stressful situations, rather than accepting your body's first response, you can take a few breaths, reset your physiology and create the time to respond with the mental clarity you need. When your exhalation is longer in proportion to your inhalation, your brain receives this as a signal that everything is OK – and lowers your stress levels accordingly.

This bomb is about to explode!

See how much you can relax your body in a single breath by extending your exhalation as much as possible in preparation for this stressful event.

How much time can you create with your exhalation?

How does this affect your next breath cycle?

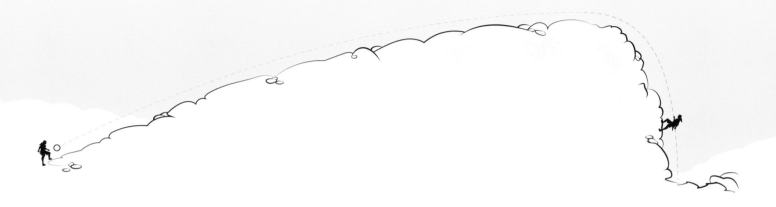

EXHILARATING EXHALE

When you combine a relaxed, slow diaphragmatic inhalation with a short and powerful exhalation, you can create a state of calm alertness without feelings of anxiety. You energize and clear the mind by filling the body with more oxygen – reducing feelings of lethargy and increasing your mental capacity for focus. This is the basic physiology behind the yogic practice of Kapalabhati, or "skull-shining breath". In Kapalabhati, calm, passive in-breaths are followed by deliberate, rhythmic, harsh exhalations through the nose, using the abdominal muscles.

This illustration requires the opposite breathing ratio to the previous page.

Take a long, calm inhalation as you help this abseiler walk leisurely up the mountain. Then, as she quickly descends the cliff face, exhale with a short, strong breath through your nose using your abdominal muscles to push the air out.

Do you feel any different?

Try a couple more breaths like this, without drawing, and notice any effects on your body, state of mind or mental clarity.

Introducing breath-drawings

For these doodling activities, place your pencil on the starting dot and become aware of the rhythm and quality of your breath for three cycles before matching the movement of your pencil to its rhythm.

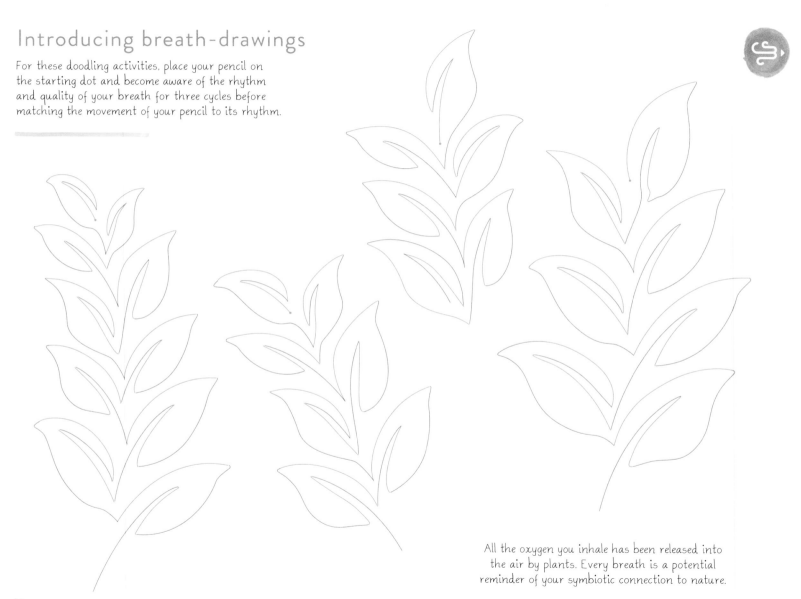

All the oxygen you inhale has been released into the air by plants. Every breath is a potential reminder of your symbiotic connection to nature.

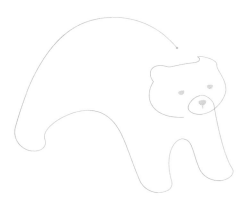

Never rush these activities - always take your time. They may take longer than you might think to complete!

Trace the breath-drawing with your finger first to give yourself an easy practice.

The more slowly and calmly you breathe, the easier and more natural these exercises become.

Some people find it helpful to count to ten for each breath cycle to pace their breathing while drawing.

Remember that during breath-drawing exercises your breath should set the pace of your pencil. Do not speed up your breathing because a line is short - slow down your pencil!

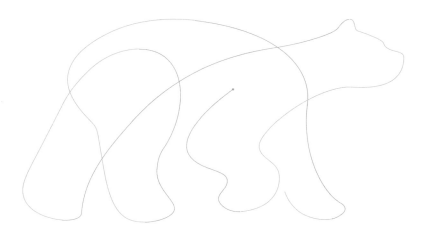

Polar bears can hold their breath for three minutes so that they can hunt underwater. It sounds like a lot... but with a little bit of practice most humans can achieve this feat!

Wanderlust

In Latin *"vagus"* means "the wanderer", and that's exactly what the vagus nerve does. Made up of over 100,000 fibres, the vagus nerve is the longest nerve in the torso, travelling down from the brain and connecting and communicating with all of your vital organs.

About 80% of the information travelling along this superhighway is the body sending signals to the brain about its current state.[3] The other 20% is the brain sending signals back down, telling the muscles and organs what to do. These signals, to and fro, control most of your homeostatic functionality as well as the relaxation response. That is to say, the vagus nerve keeps our internal systems in balance with one another.

The healthier your "vagal tone" (the strength or effectiveness of your vagus nerve), the better your body is at relaxing, recovering from states of anxiety and maintaining a state of healthy homeostasis.[4]

Advances in technology mean we can "switch on" the vagus nerve with the use of subdermal implants. These implants have been shown to greatly reduce inflammation, pain, discomfort and immobility in people suffering with chronic arthritis – such is the power of an active vagus nerve![5]

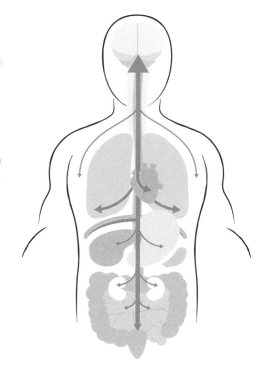

The good news, as we shall see in a few pages, is that vagal tone can be strengthened and improved without the use of technology, using simple conscious breathing techniques.

The vagus nerve stimulates your diaphragm into action. And through deep diaphragmatic breathing, you can easily and deliberately "activate" the vagus nerve, kickstarting the soothing, balancing effects of our PNS.

Tips for calm breathing to naturally boost the power of the vagus nerve:

Breathe through your nose and into your belly.

Breathe as though you are aiming the air down into your belly just below your navel, relaxing or even pushing out your abdomen to create space.

Draw down your diaphragm to inflate the lungs from the bottom up.

Let the wave of the in-breath travel up the abdomen, into the chest and all the way to your collarbone.

Exhale slowly and passively. Feel your shoulder blades relaxing down your back as the lungs naturally empty themselves.

Expel the final part of the breath using gentle pressure from your abdominal muscles. Relax the abdominal muscles and start again.

"Some doors only open from the inside. Breath is a way of accessing that door."

– Max Strom

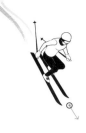

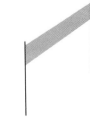

JUST LIKE GRAVITY

The more you relax, the more you begin to engage your diaphragm as you breathe, and the longer the ratio of your exhale to your inhale. When you engage the diaphragm like this, its movement naturally massages the large organs in your abdomen.

Observe your breath and notice the relaxing sensations of your exhalation.

Allowing your out-breath to become longer than your inhalations as you relax, use the ebb and flow to help this skier navigate the slalom and make her way down the mountain with smooth, easy movements.

MIND THE GAP

Pausing at the end of the out-breath lengthens
the exhalation and increases its relaxing
properties while deepening the next inhalation.
Simply drawing your attention to the natural
pause at the end of the out-breath can itself
be a very relaxing experience.

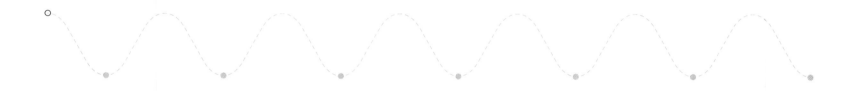

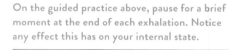

We hold a lot of tension in
our hands. Try consciously
letting your hands relax,
facing upward in a
naturally open, receiving
gesture for a few minutes.
Notice any effects this has
on the rest of your body.

Aim to grip your pencil
lightly as you do the
exercises in this book.

On the guided practice above, pause for a brief
moment at the end of each exhalation. Notice
any effect this has on your internal state.

The aim is not to hold your breath, but simply to allow
the natural pause and notice, then ride, the body's
spontaneous urge to inhale.

How does the pause affect your next inhalation?

Each pause should only last a few seconds at the most.

Relaxation is a skill. An essential
life skill. And, like all skills, it can be
learned, developed and improved.

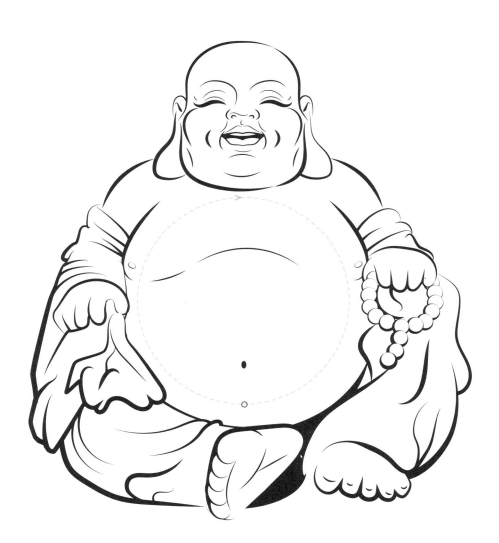

BUDDHA BELLY

Many of us feel self-conscious about our bodies and "suck in" our bellies to feel less insecure. This pattern, that we may have, at one point, adopted deliberately and self-consciously, becomes an unconscious habit. Rather than making us *look* good, it makes us *feel* bad and can really impact on our health and happiness through diminished breath quality and unnatural posture. In case you haven't heard the good news, smiling is more attractive than a flat belly! As we saw on page 12, the more you smile, the happier you are!

As you draw the circle opposite, allow your belly to relax and expand as much as you can as you inhale.

Repeat the circle a few times, feeling your belly expand a little bit more each time.

Notice how this feels. Does it feel uncomfortable to let go of your belly? If so, and you continue, are the feelings overcome by any naturally relaxing sensations?

Remember, no one is watching!

How does your heart rate?

When you breathe in, your heartbeat speeds up a tiny amount. When you breathe out, your heartbeat slows down a tiny amount. Go ahead, take a couple of breaths and see if you can notice this quirk.

The amount the heart rate fluctuates with the breath varies from person to person. It's referred to in the scientific world as "heart rate variability" (HRV). The more your heart rate fluctuates as you breathe in and out, the higher your HRV, and the more effective your autonomic nervous system – healthy fluctuation indicates that the brain is instantly aware of tiny changes in blood pressure, oxygen levels and lots of other internal factors. It is making subtle adjustments accordingly to keep the body's various internal systems in balance with one another. Most of these systems are communicating up and down the vagal pathway, so HRV is used as an accurate measurement of vagal tone. The more your heart rate fluctuates, the healthier your vagus nerve.

HRV measurement is such an accurate indicator of your overall health that it is seen as one of the most reliable predictors for all-cause mortality... i.e. how much longer you will live!

This shows just how fundamentally important healthy vagal tone and PNS response are for your overall health. If your vagal tone is low, your body's internal knowledge is low, and it isn't looking after itself as well as it could be.

Luckily, vagal tone can easily be improved with regular breathing exercises.

The power of rhythmic breathing

In their book *The Healing Power of the Breath*, Drs Patricia L. Gerbarg and Richard Brown share their groundbreaking research into how rhythmic breathing strengthens vagal tone. They call the breathing technique "coherent breathing", and it really couldn't be more simple.

The big secret?

Breathe in and out, deeply and rhythmically, at around five breaths per minute... That's in for six seconds, and out for six seconds... That's it!

This is called the "resonant rate".

Each of your internal homeostatic systems has a natural rhythm. Your breath has a rhythm, your heart rate has a rhythm, your blood pressure has a rhythm, and so on. When you breathe at a stable rate, the natural rhythms in the body begin to synchronize. Depending on your size, and health, your resonant rate will be different. For very tall people it will be around three and a half breaths per minute and for shorter people it may be as high as seven or eight breaths per minute. But for the majority, somewhere around five and six breaths per minute is optimal.[6]

After just a few seconds of this breathing technique, your heart rate will slow down and stabilize. After a few breaths, your PNS will come to life and begin to balance your homeostasis and reduce feelings of stress. After a few weeks of daily practice, the body's capacity for heart rate variability is improved... The nervous system becomes better at managing and recovering from the stress response. The immediate, positive health benefits of just one 20-minute session of coherent breathing can last up to 48 hours.[7]

Naturally, the longer you can do the practice each day, the stronger the effects. Gerbarg and Brown recommend practising for between five and twenty minutes every day. That might sound a lot, but it certainly seems like a small price to pay for reducing your risk of all-cause mortality and living a less stressed, more conscious life!

When we breathe rhythmically, our body's biorhythms begin to synchronize with the breath.

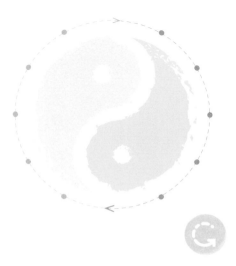

YIN AND YANG

The difference between coherent breathing and some of the other, more relaxing exercises in this book is that through equal, or near equal, inhalation and exhalation, you can balance your PNS and the SNS rather than just stimulating one or the other. This brings our nervous system into equilibrium, increasing feelings of calm alertness while decreasing feelings of tension in the body.

Complete the circle of this yin-yang illustration with equal inhalations and exhalations each lasting six seconds to balance your SNS and PNS.

Trace the circumference six times and notice how it feels to breathe this way.

PACED AND TRACED

Trace the following guided practice, pacing your breathing so that you are breathing in for five seconds and out for five seconds.

Once you have completed the illustration, put down your pencil and see if you can continue this breathing rhythm for a few minutes.

Rhythmic breathing encourages a rhythmic heart rate and, with it, rhythmic (ten-second) fluctuations in blood pressure called "Mayer waves". Recent evidence suggests that Mayer waves stimulate the release of endothelium-derived nitrous oxide (the body's home-made laughing gas!) which acts as a natural muscle relaxant and eases the tension we hold in our muscles, particularly in the walls of our heart and blood vessels.[8]

In the free space above experiment with some different ratios, 4:4, 4:6, 6:6, and so on, and see what feels comfortable for you.

BREATH COUNTING

There are four potential breathing moments we can control when breath counting:

1. Inhalation

2. Hold

3. Exhalation

4. Pause

Depending on the length of each phase, relative to the others, a different effect is created on the body and mind. The longer the out-breath, the greater the stimulation of the PNS, and therefore the more relaxing. Meanwhile, the more equal the inhalation and the exhalation, the more balanced the SNS and the PNS. Holding the breath for a brief period at the top of the inhalation oxygenates the blood and increases energy levels.

Trace your pencil along the dotted lines. **The distance from one dot to the next should last roughly one second.**

How does each different pattern affect your body?

What about your mind?

Holding the breath can feel unnatural and awkward at first, but once you create a rhythm, it will feel more comfortable. Counting the breath gives you something to focus the mind on, which helps if you're easily distracted during normal breathing exercises. It also acts like a mantra, taking up headspace that might otherwise be occupied by negative thoughts.

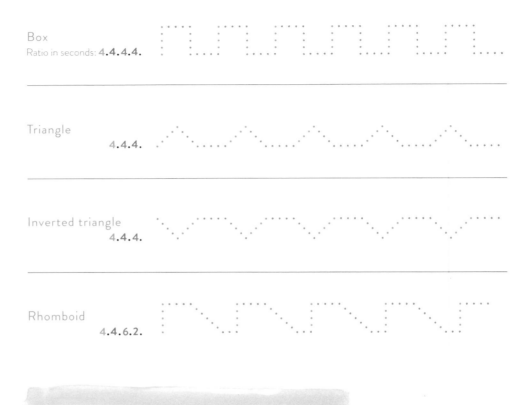

Box
Ratio in seconds: **4.4.4.4.**

Triangle
4.4.4.

Inverted triangle
4.4.4.

Rhomboid
4.4.6.2.

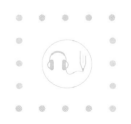

"Box breathing" was developed by well-being educator and ex-marine commander Mark Divine. It is now taught to the American military as a tool that soldiers can use to keep their cool in stressful, life-threatening situations.

Extended versions of these meditations are available at **drawbreath.com**

BREATHING "PATTERN"

Using the techniques explained on the opposite page, experiment and create your own repeated breathing patterns.

Vary your holds and pauses to create your own shapes.

Take one second to travel between each dot.

You may wish to draw a shape first and then guide your finger around it in time with the breath.

What effect does your pattern have on your body and mind?

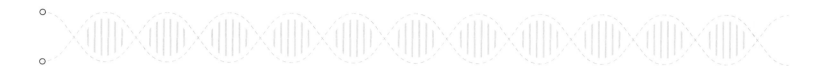

OXYGEN IS ANTI-AGING

Not only does chronic stress increase your risk of heart disease and other health issues[9], it slowly degrades your DNA, speeding up the aging process[10].

Each strand of your DNA has a protective tip called a telomere. Like the plastic cap on the end of a shoelace, telomeres keep the strands of DNA from becoming damaged and frayed. Telomeres protect the DNA from premature aging, so the quality of your telomeres is a good indicator of your actual biological age. The healthier your telomeres, the healthier you feel (and the younger you look!).

Stress harms your telomeres, but a calm physiological state helps to repair them.

Not only can you reduce the damage to your telomeres through breathing practices, you can actually reverse it and turn back the clock on your biological age![11]

Use rhythmic breathing to balance your internal nervous system and "strengthen" these strands of DNA.

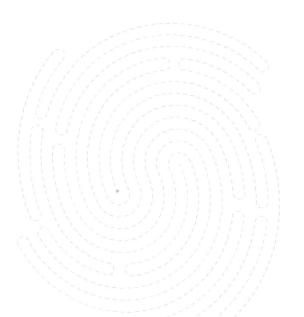

YOUR BREATHING IDENTITY

Like a fingerprint, each person's breathing pattern is unique to them. A combination of all of the varying factors we discussed on pages 18 and 19 come together to tell a one-off story about that person's life and how they are feeling in this moment.

Use the natural rhythm of your own breath to trace this fingerprint illustration.

Remember, you are observing the breath and following its pattern, so let the natural rate of your breath draw your pencil across the page. Allow the unique ebb and flow of your breath control its speed.

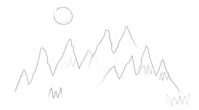

PEAK EXPERIENCE

Getting the most out of your breath helps
you to get the most out of your life.

Use the simple free-breathing patterns you
have learned so far to draw a peaceful mountain
range using the patterns of your breath.

Feeling emotional

The breath can give us insight into how we are feeling, even when we are not aware of it. When we are anxious, stressed or even very focused, we tighten our bodies and our breath becomes shallow. When we are relaxed, so is our breathing.

Each emotion has its own breathing pattern. These are most noticeable at the extremes, when we are laughing or crying. But we also "wait with bated breath" in moments of anxiety and expectation. Or "sigh a breath of relief" when feeling... relief.

If you imitate the breathing pattern associated with an emotion, it won't take long before you actually begin to feel that emotion. As we saw earlier, the mind-body system is a two-way street.

How we feel affects how we breathe. But how we breathe affects how we feel!

Our emotion affects not just our breathing but our posture; when we are feeling threatened or defeated, we will hang our heads and slump our shoulders in the exact opposite way to someone who has just won a gold medal at the Olympics. This posture closes our chest space and has a negative impact on our breathing – a negative cycle is created.

To breathe deeply, to our full potential, we must assume a positive posture, and a positive cycle is created.

MIND READER

Use this page to draw someone else's breath... Perhaps someone you know, or, if you're feeling adventurous, a stranger you're sat opposite on public transport or nearby in a café.

Fold the page corner over these instructions so they don't have to know what you are doing!

Listen to the sound of their breathing and sneakily observe the movements of their body to workout *where* they breathe.

What muscles are they using? What is their ratio? How deep is their breath? How is their breath affecting their posture? How is their posture affecting their breath?

What impression does the resulting picture give you of the person? What can you tell about their emotional state from their breathing pattern?

Vive la résistance!

Softly restricting your breath by creating subtle resistance slows down your exhalation and creates gentle pressure in the lungs. Both of these factors activate the PNS. The conscious control and increased pressure strengthen your muscles, making you a more effective breather and protecting you from injury.[12]

Opting to breathe through the nose rather than the mouth is the simplest form of resistance breathing.

Nose breathing also has other benefits. Organic, spiralling pathways in the nasal cavity heat or cool the air as needed, while fine hairs and mucus membranes filter the air, acting as a natural defence protecting the lungs from harmful dust and bacteria.

BLOW BUBBLES

Purse your lips as you exhale and blow slowly and smoothly, as though you are carefully blowing bubbles.

Inhaling through the nose and exhaling through pursed lips, draw bubbles to complete this illustration using the circle technique we learned on page 40.

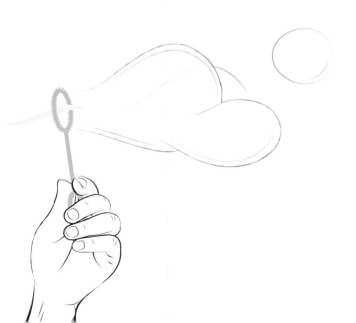

OCEAN BREATHING

Ujjayi breath (pronounced oo-jai), sometimes called "ocean breathing", is the yogic practice of creating resistance at the back of the throat while breathing through your nose.

Inhale through your nose. Open your mouth and breathe out as though you are fogging up a mirror, then, without stopping your exhalation, close your mouth. Notice how the breath now comes out of your nose, making a soft sound? Retain this resistance in your throat to create the same, slightly quieter, sound on your next inhalation. This subtle resistance is ujjayi breathing.

The sound should be soft, like a baby snoring or peaceful waves lapping the shore.

Practice ujjayi breathing through your nose while drawing the waves lapping on this shoreline.

See if you can match the sound of your pencil moving across the page with the sound of your inhalation and exhalation.

The purpose is to create delicate resistance, naturally drawing your attention to and lengthening the breath cycle. Making rough snoring sounds like a chainsaw won't be relaxing and can damage the delicate membranes in your nose.

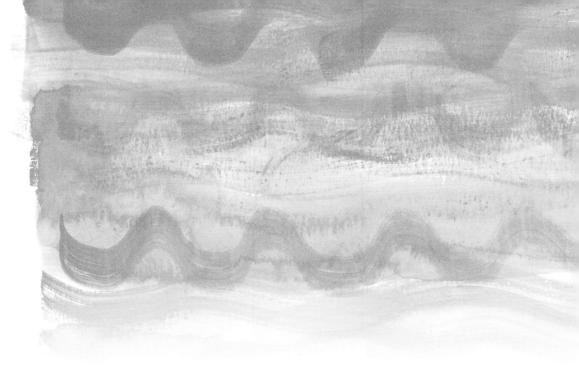

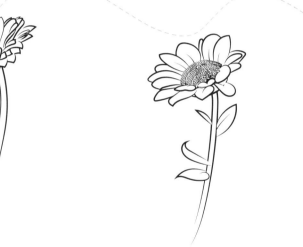

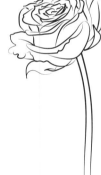

GOOD VIBES

Singing, chanting and humming are all forms of resistance breathing. You create sound in your throat by tightening your vocal chords and restricting the flow of air. As well as creating naturally soothing vibrations, these activities cause you to simultaneously slow down your breath rate and increase the ratio of your exhalation; two alterations to our breathing pattern that stimulate the PNS.

Help this bumblebee have a smooth landing on each of these flowers by humming a low note on your exhalation, making it naturally smoother and longer.

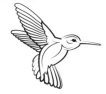

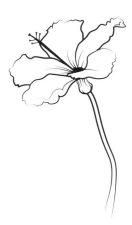

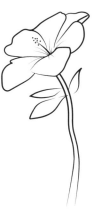

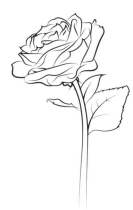

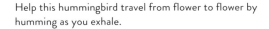

Help this hummingbird travel from flower to flower by humming as you exhale.

During vibrational breathing exercises, sounds travel down the body and cause your organs to vibrate. See if you can feel the vibrations in your extremities, your shoulders, elbows, forearms and fingers. What about your feet? The lower the tone of your hum, the further the vibrations will travel.

When we're stressed, we unconsciously prioritize our inhalations. This is the body preparing us to run away from threats. But when we're stressed *all the time*, breathing like this means the muscles we use to exhale become weaker. Resistance and vibrational breathing exercises strengthen these muscles with slow controlled exhalations.

This makes a lot of sense

We generally think of ourselves as having five senses: vision, hearing, smell, taste and touch. You were probably taught that these are your senses in primary school.

In fact, this list of senses is woefully inadequate. We can be said to have more than a dozen senses that contribute to our conscious experience. Our bodies sense our blood pressure through stretch receptors in our blood vessels. We measure our oxygen and carbon dioxide levels through chemoreceptors in our brains. Our muscles moving beneath our skin give us information about how tense they are, how stretched they are. We have a sense called "proprioception" that tells us what position our body is in, without having to look.

What about our sense of balance? Or time? Or our levels of energy? These senses are, at first glance, amorphous, constantly shifting and overlapping. We take them for granted, and rarely think about them, but you would feel very strange if all of a sudden you couldn't feel these elements of your experience.

> The more connected we feel to our hearts and our gut feelings, the stronger our intuition.

Notice that the five traditional senses all refer to how we interact with the outside world.

Meanwhile, the traditionally ignored senses are all to do with our bodily, internal world. We have a cultural bias toward seeing ourselves as separate from the world; the world is something "outside" us that we are separated from, and interact with, through our skin. To borrow an analogy from philosopher Alan Watts: we see ourselves as coming "into" the world as outsiders or tourists, instead of coming "out" of the world like fruit to a tree, even though the latter is more accurate.

Four out of the five traditionally recognized senses are located exclusively in our heads, which supports the illusion that we, our "selves", are located somewhere above the neck, in the brain. But the truth trickles into our everyday language... We talk about having "gut feelings" and speaking "from the heart". We know deep down that our minds don't end at our brain stem. We are "embodied" minds.

In the scientific world the sum of these inner feelings is referred to as "interoception".

INNER KNOWLEDGE

Take a moment to look inside yourself. Can you feel your heart beating in your chest?

Take five relaxed diaphragmatic breaths, counting to five on the inhale and six on the exhale.

Can you feel your heartbeat now?

Many people report noticing their heart beat much more clearly after just a few minutes of slow, deep, conscious breathing.

This simple exercise is an immediate, consciously experienced example of how diaphragmatic breathing strengthens our interoceptive abilities and connects us with our internal lives by "lighting up" the vagus nerve.

Slow, deep breathing activates the PNS – the vagus nerve "wakes up" and the channels of perception into our own bodies become clearer, like a radio being tuned to the correct frequency. Almost immediately, our body becomes more effective at regulating its own internal homeostasis. Extended periods of breathing like this are shown to reduce over-zealous autoimmune responses like inflammation.[13]

The bad news is that a diminished capacity for interoception is related to many psychophysiological disorders like hypertension, as well as anxiety and depression.[14] Feeling disconnected from our bodies in this way not only stops the body from functioning properly, it even weakens our experience of empathy, making us feel disconnected from other people and the world at large.

The good news is, we can do something about it. Internal sensitivity can be trained and improved with conscious focus and breathing practice. By focusing on our internal states, we can increase the body's natural capacity for interoception, improving its inner knowledge, making it more effective at maintaining its own equilibrium, connecting us to our intuition and improving our overall health.

ONE-HANDED MEDITATION

Place your non-drawing hand onto the page so that all of your fingers and your thumb are in contact with the paper.

Starting at the base of your little finger, draw around the contour of your hand. Breathe in as you ascend, and out as you descend around each finger, allowing your breath volume to naturally increase as the size of your fingers increases and finishing with a long exhale from the tip of your thumb to your wrist.

Now place your hand on the table next to the book. Take a few moments to notice what the surface feels like under your palm, and the feeling (or lack of feeling) of air over the top of your hand.

Move your focus inside your hand and see how many of the internal senses you can feel. Can you feel the movement and tension of your muscles? Your heartbeat? Your energy levels? It may help to close your eyes. What sensations do you feel that let you know your hand is still there?

Draw the patterns of these movements of energy as abstract lines and shapes inside the hand outline you have just created.

Remember, the deeper and slower your breathing, the stronger your internal feelings will be.

After completing this exercise, slowly expand your awareness, from your hand, up your arm and into the rest of your body. What feelings are there that you hadn't noticed before? It is amazing how capable we are of ignoring our inner body sensations most of the time.

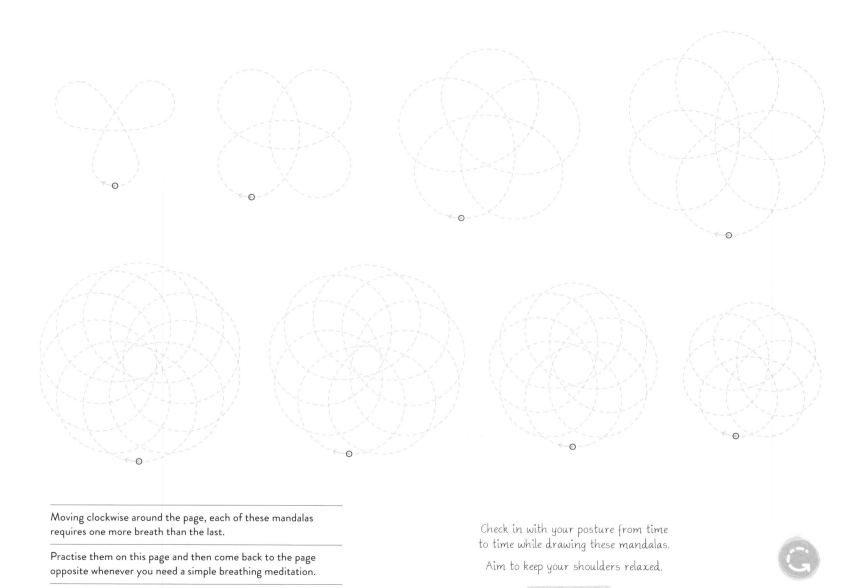

Moving clockwise around the page, each of these mandalas requires one more breath than the last.

Practise them on this page and then come back to the page opposite whenever you need a simple breathing meditation.

Check in with your posture from time to time while drawing these mandalas.

Aim to keep your shoulders relaxed.

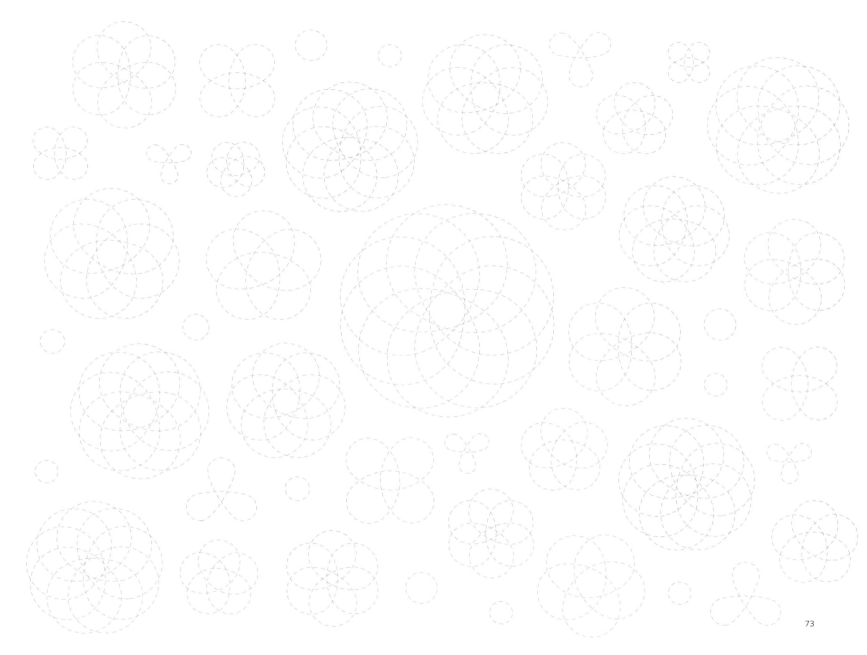

Right is wrong

Nestled in the middle of your brain is the part called the insula (it's "insula"-ted by the rest of the brain.)

The insula is the centre of your interoceptive experience; the hub of your "inner" self. All of your moment-to-moment internal experience, the sensations of your inner body, from taste, to emotions, to your experience of time, and even your model for feeling other people's emotions and experiences, pass through the insula. This is where your perceptive model of your inner world is formed and experienced. [15]

The insula is divided into two halves which correspond to positive and negative experiences. When your experience is negative or unpleasant, for example, when you experience pain, the right side of the insula is more active. And when you are happy or experiencing pleasant sensations, the left side lights up with activity. [16]

Give yourself a breather

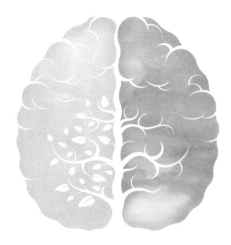

Put simply, the right side of the insula is for experiencing challenges, while the left side is for stimulating feelings of rest and reward. The sides are, roughly speaking, binary. When one side is activated, it suppresses activity in the other side. So, by activating the left side, we can effectively "switch off" activity in the right side.

The sensory nerves in your lungs and heart that are stimulated by breathing slowly and deeply ("bronchopulmonary afferents", if you want to be really geeky about it) are entirely vagal and parasympathetic. They run information from the lower lungs and diaphragm up the vagus nerve, through the heart and directly into the left side of your insula, where they instantly stimulate neural activity. This creates immediate positive feelings and, by suppressing the activity of the right insula, can even create a measurable decrease in pain sensitivity. [17]

This shift in activity, from right to left, nudges your default perception of your internal state from negative to positive...

... through deep diaphragmatic breathing, you can switch the setting of how you experience the world from negative to positive.

Rhythmic, slow breathing acts like a bellows that blows out the negative and feeds the warm embers of positive emotion and empathic sensitivity deep in our brains.

Down is up

The further down in your abdomen you breathe, the more you stimulate the uplifting activity of the left insula.

BODIES CAN BODY SCAN

Close your eyes and observe the feelings in your body as though you are in an art gallery, stepping back and viewing a work of art... What grabs your attention? Are there areas of vibrancy? Or beauty?

Are there feelings of energy and movement within your body? Swirling patterns? Warm or cool areas?

Can you feel your pulse in each area of your body?

Let your attention rest on each area; see if it *feels* a certain colour, or if a particular shape or pattern comes to mind.

Methodically scan your body, moving your focus from the tips of your toes to the top of your head and translate the sensations into colours and patterns on this body-shaped canvas as though it is a mirror that shows your inner sensations.

Don't be afraid to revisit areas and layer your image with multiple mediums.

I recommend including coloured highlighter pens for this exercise to create broad, vibrant strokes.

After completing your picture, you may wish to consult page 124 to see how close you are to the traditional colours associated with yogic chakras!

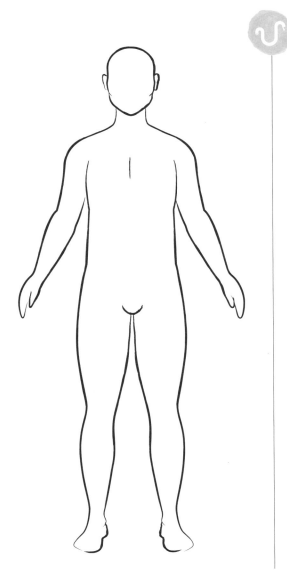

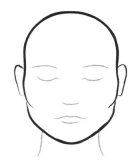

FACE FACTS

Since long before we could talk, we have been using our faces to communicate how we are feeling. They reflect our internal emotions without us realizing. So most of us hold a lot of tension in our jaws, eyebrows, forehead and temples.

Do you frown when you're reading? Or scrunch your face up in concentration while you draw? If so, what effect does this have on your body and mind?

Relaxing your face sends signals from your body that relax your mind.

As you colour in this face shape, imagine the colour on the page corresponding to relaxing energy filling that area of your face.

Colour in one area at a time: both cheeks, both eyebrows and so on. Colour in your eyes last of all.

You may wish to use cool or warm colours to soothe or relax areas of tension.

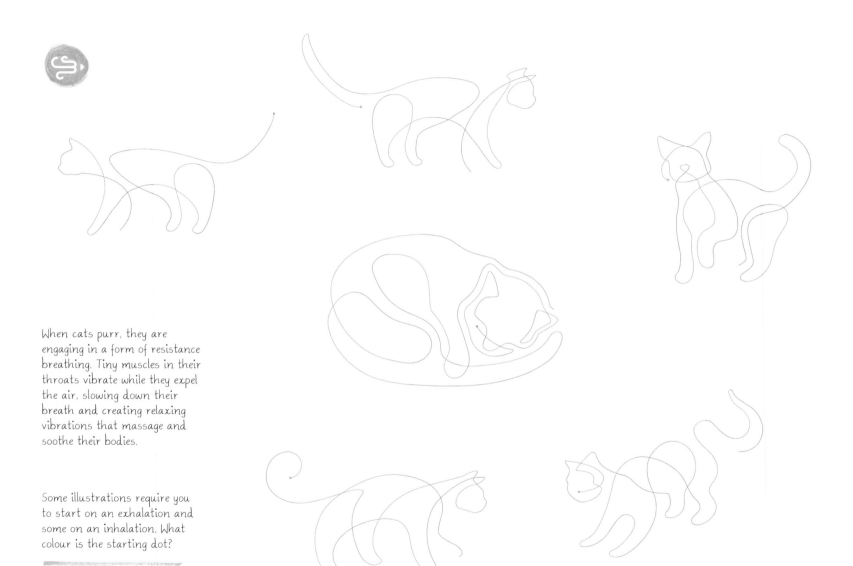

When cats purr, they are engaging in a form of resistance breathing. Tiny muscles in their throats vibrate while they expel the air, slowing down their breath and creating relaxing vibrations that massage and soothe their bodies.

Some illustrations require you to start on an exhalation and some on an inhalation. What colour is the starting dot?

When did you forget how to breathe?

If you observe a child running, playing or at rest, you will notice that they intuitively breathe into their bellies.

When we are babies, we use our whole bodies to breathe. But as teenagers, we become self-conscious of our bodies and begin to hold our bellies in. As adults we hold on to stressful experiences as tension in our muscles on an unconscious level. Over time this tension accumulates, and our breathing becomes increasingly constricted.

By the time most of us are in our early twenties, we have lost the natural ease and rhythm of the breath. Once we are adults, many of us breathe exclusively into our upper chests.

Children not only breathe better, they are naturally more present in each moment. They live in the now, quickly letting go of positive and negative emotions as they pass through them. One minute they are crying, the next they are laughing. Each day is fresh. As a result they live in a natural state of curiosity; they are distracted by everyday things and become completely absorbed in the most mundane of tasks. They live half-submerged in a world of imagination, making creative play easy and exhilarating. Once again, we see that the journey of the mind and the body are deeply entwined.

The next part of the book explores some ways of regaining childlike curiosity, focus and happiness using the breath.

"The wise man is a happy child."

– Arnaud Desjardins

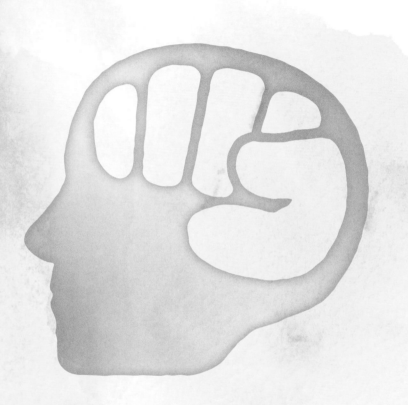

PART 2

MIND

The secret to Zen?

... Be "now", not "then"

"Breath
is the link
between
mind and
body."

— Dan Brulé

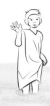

Everything flows

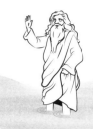

Change is the only constant in life. This was the observation made by the ancient Greek philosopher Heraclitus. Everything is transient, ever-changing, impermanent, temporary. All of Being is moving and shifting in a constant state of flux, from one moment to the next. The idea is best captured in his famous maxim *"You can never step in the same river twice."*

Heraclitus was mainly talking about the physical world, but the same is true for our experience of consciousness – our mental lives. The world around us is constantly changing, and so are our thoughts and perceptions.

At around the same time, in the fifth century BCE, another deep thinker was making similar observations 6,000 miles away in the foothills of the Himalayas. Siddhartha Gautama, who would later become known as the Buddha, had been rocked as a young man by the realization that human life is subject to impermanence; we age, we get sick, we die. As a result, he dedicated his life to finding liberation from what he saw as an endless cycle of discontentment.

The concept that the Greek philosophers had called "flux", the Buddhists would name *"anicca"*, meaning "impermanence".

They label it as one of the three unalterable facts about existence, the other two being that we are, bound to suffer *(dukkha)* and that our idea of our "self" is an illusion *(anatta)*.

This all might sound pessimistic at first, but the insight can be liberating. It helps us to understand the nature of suffering – it is because things are impermanent that attachment leads to suffering. It is not impermanence that is the problem – it is attachment.

Clinging to material possessions, mental states, times in our past and even the present moment causes us to experience fear, anxiety and disappointment. Attachment to things is unwise if we know nothing is permanent.

Things can only be appreciated as they are experienced in the moment. Not as they were in the past, or might be in the future, or how we think they "should" be. We can only feel truly whole in "the now".

Using the shifting ebb and flow of your breath as a guide, draw a river flowing across this page connecting the young boy and the old man.

Draw a few leisurely, overlapping lines.

Colour in the shapes made by the overlapping lines to complete your drawing.

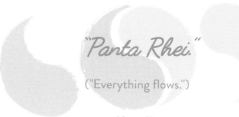

"Panta Rhei."

("Everything flows.")

– Heraclitus

"How can the past and future be, when the past no longer is, and the future is not yet?

As for the present, if it were always present and never moved on to become the past, it would not be time, it would be eternity."

– St Augustine of Hippo,
Confessions Book 11

When St Augustine wrote these words in 400 CE, he became the first Western philosopher to describe their subjective experience as a fundamental account of reality. His description more truthfully reflects our *experience* of time than do our "common sense" *ideas about* time…

… The past and future exist only in the mind; even the present moment only exists as "time" once it has become "the past".

It sounds complicated, but his point was simple – time exists only as an idea. The present is our only reality.

His insight was largely overlooked until the eighteenth-century philosopher Immanuel Kant reminded us that *"Time exists only in the relations between perceptions."* Later, in the twentieth century, Bertrand Russell called Augustine's observations *"a great advance"* for Western philosophy, but they have never really been put into practice in the West.

This isn't just wordplay to entertain armchair philosophers; these sages had stumbled onto something important, something with a real, practical application. Something that meditators in the East had known for millennia… The past and future exist only as ideas in our minds, yet we worry about the past, and we fret about the future, and as a result we miss the present moment – we miss what's real.

If we allow this pattern to continue, we spend our entire lives looking backward, or forward, and we miss the whole thing!

No academic has put it better than the American cartoonist Bil Keane who reminds us: *"Yesterday is the past, tomorrow is the future, but today is a gift. That's why it's called 'the present'."*

Regretting in past tense…

… fretting in future tense…

… (no wonder we're so tense)

THINKING STRAIGHT

Place the tip of your pencil on the starting point at the bottom of the "present" column.

Without moving your pencil, take a few moments to focus on the moment-to-moment sensations of your breathing – take your time.

Each time you find your attention has wandered from the experience of your breath and into thinking, observe where it has gone.

Think about the thought: is it about the past? ... Or the future?

Once you have labelled your thought, drag your pencil up and across to the dot in the corresponding column to record where your mind has gone. Then pull it back into the "present" column.

Focus your attention back on your breathing and repeat the process until you have been distracted by thoughts six times (and reached the top of the grid).

How long did it take for your mind to drift?

Where did it go? Were you thinking more about the past or the future? How accurate were your thoughts?

If your thoughts are judgements about the present, for example, "What a stupid exercise, this is a waste of time", wait for the next thought, "I should never have wasted money on this book" (past), or the next, "I should go and do the washing-up instead" (future).

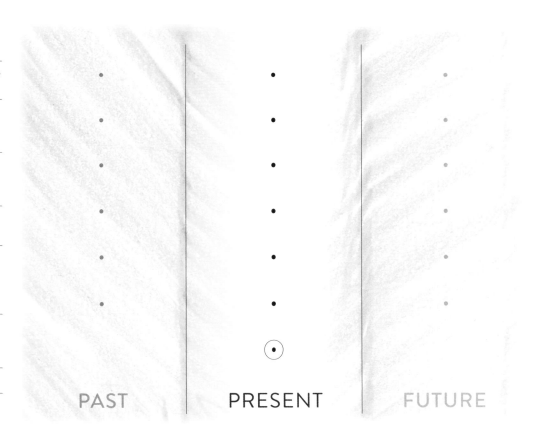

PAST   PRESENT   FUTURE

This exercise creates a crude map of our experience of time. It shows us how easy it is for our consciousness to be pulled away from the present and into rumination about simplified and biased versions of our past, or imagined, projected versions of our future.

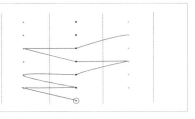

An extended version of this meditation is available at drawbreath.com

It takes two

You have two selves. Two ways of being.

Your experiencing self, the self who answers the question, "Are you enjoying that sandwich?" and the storytelling self, the self who answers the question, "Did you enjoy that sandwich?"

The storytelling self is completely verbal and based in the abstract and the imagined; the past and the future. Meanwhile, the experiencing self, by definition, is based in the present; in reality.

We see our lives through the filter of the storytelling self, and we try to fit each day and new experience into its narrative. This is limiting. We want our story to have meaning or to be impressive. We want to tell a story that makes sense, and, therefore, often without realizing it, we are prone to simplification, bias and embellishment.

According to recent studies, our minds tend to wander around 50% of the time, and 60% of our distracted thoughts are negative.[18,19]

This means we are wasting more than a quarter of our waking lives, an average of four hours a day, absorbed in negative self-talk.

So how do we live more in "the now"?

Repeating a negative story about our lives over and over in our heads creates feelings of low self-worth. But even telling a positive, coherent story can create tension and unhappiness in the present.

Telling ourselves a positive story generates momentary pleasure, but it also causes attachment; we don't want to lose the story, or for anyone to challenge it. And so, this story, that no one else cares about or even hears, except ourselves, becomes an object of anxiety. It's like carrying around an expensive and delicate jewel that we could break or lose at any moment.

Negative thoughts can cause a negative mind-to-body interaction... All of this mental stuff, happening invisibly, somewhere above the neck, impacts on the body.

The prefrontal lobe (the part of the brain where our abstract thoughts get turned into words that only we can hear) is brand new in evolutionary terms. Its ancient older sibling, the amygdala (the part that pushes the fight-or-flight button), can't tell the difference between what the experiencing self is seeing ("Mmm, a sandwich!") and the thoughts that the prefrontal lobe is broadcasting ("I wonder if this sandwich will make me fat? I've put on so much weight recently, no one will ever love me. At least I have this sandwich. Oh, it's gone. Maybe I should order another sandwich.").

Identifying with the storytelling part of ourselves (in other words, listening to thoughts all day and taking them seriously) takes up most of our awareness and stops us from having access to the new experiences happening right in front of us.

Our thoughts about reality are in the way of reality.

The storytelling self is always talking about the past or the future. It takes us away from the here and now.

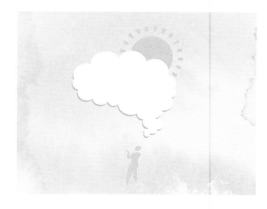

We are not the only animal with an amygdala. But we are the only animal with a prefrontal lobe that can create advanced language, and, therefore, we're the only creature that has the ability to constantly misfire its fight-or-flight response by telling itself an inaudible, and sometimes terrifying, story about the world (a story that rarely has any bearing on the actual world).

Events →

Year →

PUT YOUR LIFE ON THE LINE

Add years to the line above to create a timeline of your life. Mark a few key events in your life on your timeline.

Perhaps note down your career history, or the places you have lived. Include some key friendships and first times. Make a little note of whether the experience was positive or negative.

Were you aware of the experience of writing about yourself? Your pen moving across the page, the colour of the ink? The room around you? Or were you completely absorbed in the story?

How often do you taste your food while you are eating it? Most of the time we only taste the first few bites before we are distracted by thoughts and lose ourselves in storytelling.

So how do we live more in the "now"?

The solution is simple (at least in writing).

> – Learn to focus on your direct experience rather than your thoughts about it.

Not only does this mode of being increase the availability of new experiences, it gives us a new perspective on the importance of thoughts. Ordinarily central to our consciousness, they become just another part of our experience that we can choose whether or not to pay attention to. We embrace a state in which we can expand our awareness to include our hearts, our gut feelings and the wider world.

Focusing repeatedly on the breath trains you to direct your awareness toward your experience of your body, strengthening the neural and nervous pathways of the "experiencing self".

Focusing on experience when we are in rest-and-digest mode is especially rewarding. Our somatic experience is more positive than usual, and this creates a positive body-to-mind interaction.

> **"When we bring our mind into our body, the body becomes mindful, and the mind becomes embodied."**
>
> – Donna Farhi

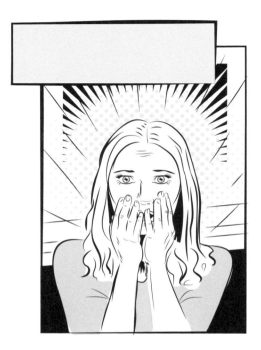

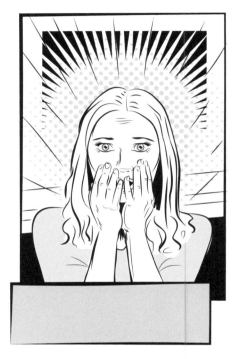

REFRAMING

Thoughts are like the descriptive text that sits in a little box just outside of a comic strip. They can change, and everything inside the frame changes... without the picture changing at all.

Your thoughts about reality are not reality, they are just descriptions of it.

They are the lyrics, not the music.
The menu, not the meal.

Write captions in the boxes above that let each image tell a completely different story.

Share your creations online #**DrawBreathBook**

You wouldn't give a speech without clearing your throat. So why do you think without clearing your mind?

LOST IN THOUGHT

You can't out-think your own thoughts...

If you're stuck in a negative thought pattern, *more thinking* won't stop it. But rumination is only one of the many mental states available to you. By expanding your awareness beyond just your thoughts, moving it deeper into your body or to the outside world, and exploring other parts of your available experience, you can break the pattern of negative thinking.

Help this thinker escape the maze of their thinking pattern and expand their attention toward the rest of their inner-body experience.

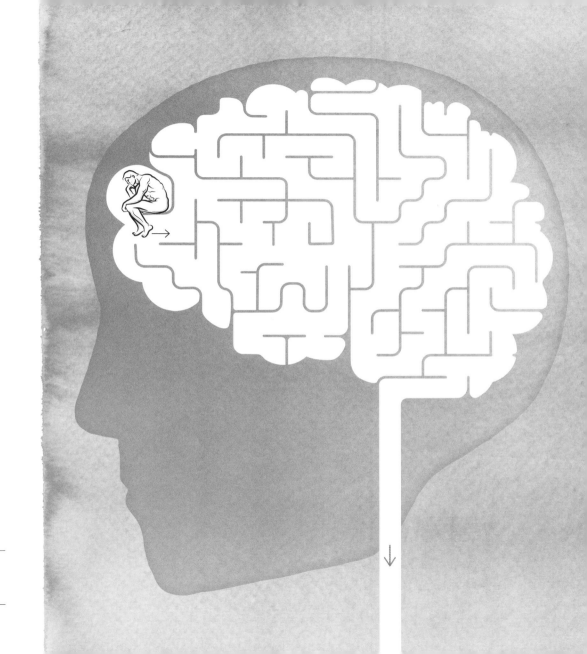

Mind full?

... time to be mindful.

Try not to think of anything for as long as you can.

Clear your mind entirely and don't think any thoughts whatsoever.

Go!

How long did you last? Most of us can only manage a few moments at most.

Even when we try our hardest, it's nearly impossible not to think thoughts! We quickly lose our focus and the mind naturally wanders.

Thinking is natural, normal and often useful and enjoyable, but when we find ourselves repeatedly drawn into rumination about the past or anxiety about the future it is helpful to *think about thoughts* in a new way.

The exercise above illustrates that most thoughts are something that happen to you, something you listen to... not always something you control. They are just another part of your available experience, like sights and sounds. Thoughts are your mind offering you possible interpretations of the world, rather than your own true internal voice.

Rather than trying not to think, try actively listening to your next few thoughts. Observe your mind as it wanders for just a few seconds.

When we start to become deliberately conscious of our thoughts in this way, we can begin to notice when they trigger negative physical or emotional responses – responses that, in turn, trigger more stressful thoughts and create a negative cycle between the mind and body.

Once we notice this distinction and recognize the patterns of thought and emotion, our negative thoughts begin to lose their power over us. We begin to see them as transient, temporary, optional ways of interpreting the world instead of as true, solid reflections of reality.

Thoughts are often in the way of our direct experience of the moment. When we don't take them at face value, when we expand our attention to include other parts of our awareness with purpose and acceptance – we experience peace.

Mindfulness is the act of paying attention to the present moment with curiosity, kindness, compassion and acceptance. And it starts with focusing on the breath.

When we stop being distracted by our thoughts and shift our focus inward toward our bodily sensations, or outward to the world around us, we become more present. We start to notice life's immediate pleasures as they unfold instead of missing them, absorbed in thinking mode. This has enormous knock-on effects for our mental and physical well-being.

By training our attention and exploring our awareness with repeated meditation practice, we can build our capacity for mental focus and tranquillity. Our responses to whatever we may experience in life become more measured and less reactive.

By paying deliberate attention like this, we increase our awareness of our thoughts, feelings and actions as well as our understanding of our attention itself. Practising this skill strengthens our ability to notice, meet and respond to life's challenges with a clear and open mind, improved resilience and renewed focus.

Mindfulness is an experiential process. To experience the benefits, you have to engage with the practice.

In people who meditate regularly, there is visible growth in the parts of the brain that relate to empathy. Observing our own minds and bodies improves our ability to empathize, understand and connect with other people.[20]

*Go to **drawbreath.com** to try a guided audio mindfulness meditation*

*"One conscious breath
... in and out...
is a meditation."*

– Eckhart Tolle

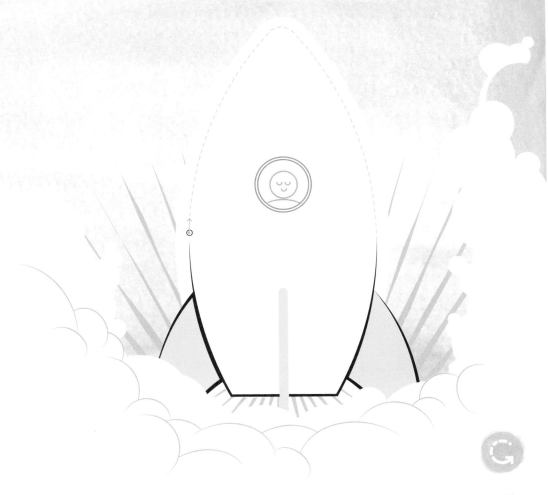

READY FOR LAUNCH

Pay close attention to the natural texture of your breath as you draw **one** slow breath on this page. Listen to its sounds and feel its sensations as you complete this drawing of a rocket.

Put your pencil down and pay exactly the same amount of attention to every moment of your next breath **without drawing it**.

See how many breaths in a row you can study like this. If your mind wanders, just bring it back to the breath and begin again.

You may find your breath automatically slows and expands as you observe it; this is natural.

This is meditation.

MIND OVER NATTER

Formal mindfulness meditation involves sitting (or lying down) and drawing your attention to the naturally grounding sensations of your feet touching the floor and your bum supported by the seat, then on to the organic, inner sensations of the breath. And finally, expanding your awareness to include your other inner feelings, thoughts and the world around you.

Meditation isn't intended to **stop** thoughts. It's a way of stepping back from them and widening the focus of our awareness to include the other elements of our experience.

The mind naturally wanders. The practice of meditation is to notice when it has and bring your attention back from the thought, to the sensations of the breath.

Thoughts arise and pass, lasting only a moment...

... roughly one breath.

Using the rhythm of your breath, draw the path of a thought as it enters and leaves this person's consciousness.

The tip of your pencil is the tipping point between past and future as they slip from one into the other on the page.

The pencil point is always now; its graphite wake is the past, the blank page its future.

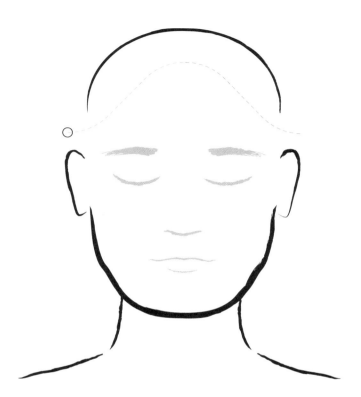

Notice each moment at a moment's notice

On average, we perceive moments as only a few seconds long before our minds move on, reset and begin to change focus and interpretation. This just so happens to be around the time it takes us to breathe out.

SCHOOL OF THOUGHT

Our thoughts and impressions continuously change, appearing and disappearing as one moment passes into another… but the breath is always there.

Take your time to trace the rhythm of the breath up and down across this page at your own pace and notice how many different mental events cross your mind's eye and disappear.

Don't attach yourself to them, just observe them come and go and centre your attention back on your breath.

Be compassionate to your own feelings and do not judge yourself when you realize you have become distracted. It is the point of meditation to notice when you have drifted back into thinking mode, so that you can practise shifting back into experiencing mode. When you do turn your attention to thoughts, aim to observe them as though they are something you are listening to; just another part of your experience, rather than something you are doing.

You may find, when you try to focus your awareness on your thoughts, they become very shy. It is difficult to hold one down and study it without it disappearing!

The Witness

If you can hear your thoughts, who is listening?

When you begin to eavesdrop on your thoughts impartially, observing them as they enter and leave your mind, instead of identifying with them, you realize that you are not the thinker, you are the listener – the spectator in your own mind. There is a thinking self and a listening "Self" – a speaker and a witness. The witness is your truer, deeper Self. Consciousness. The real You.

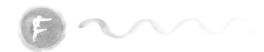

Switching frequencies

Imagine your conscious experience as a radio. Your awareness is the signal. There are thousands of wavelengths passing through the radio. Every area of your body, your senses, your thoughts, emotions and feelings are all different frequencies that are available for you to tune in to at any time. What station are you usually listening to? For most people, it's a talk show where they are the only caller, calling in and discussing their problems with a presenter who also happens to be themselves.

Is it time to change what's playing?

Meditation helps us to practise shifting our awareness; tuning in to vibrations in our bodies that we usually ignore completely. Through training our attention, we fine-tune our ability to change and improve signal input and listen to the music of our bodies and the world around us.

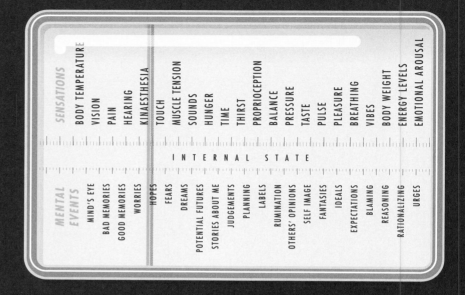

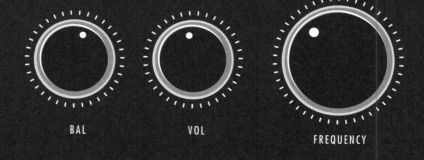

BAL   VOL   FREQUENCY

CHANGE YOUR TUNE

For five successive breaths, draw your attention to the sensations of air passing into and out of your nose. Notice the temperature of the air. For the last few breaths, notice any subtle smells in the environment.

Notice the sounds of the next few breaths. How is each different from the last? How is each unique? As you continue, expand your awareness to sounds inside the room, and then outside it. What's the furthest sound you can hear?

Observe your visual field as you draw. Notice the unique textures in the path of the graphite. Are there colours or textures on the back of your hand that you've never noticed before? How is the quality of the light in the room? Finally, expand your visual awareness to your peripheral vision.

Feel the sensations of your feet touching the floor, your clothes resting against your body and the movement of your hand against the paper. Can you feel the vibrations of resistance through your pencil?

For the next five breaths let your attention rest on the content of your mind. What is crossing your mind's eye? Are there thoughts or feelings that you can be aware of? See if you can catch a thought as it occurs. Where did it come from? Can you watch it go?

This exercise hardly scratches the surface of the available experience you can explore using the breath as an anchor! Pick another channel from the "sensations" frequencies on the radio opposite and focus on it for five breaths. What's on the aiwaves?

RADIO ME

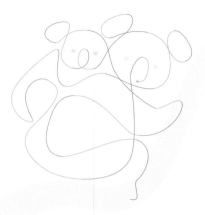

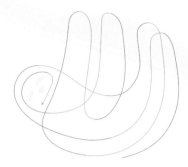

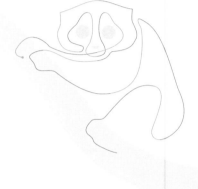

Modern life moves fast.
Sometimes, slowing
down actually gives
you more time.

Slow down your breathing
and give yourself more
time to trace these
slow animals.

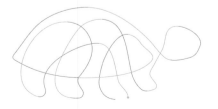

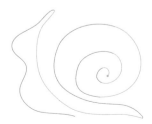

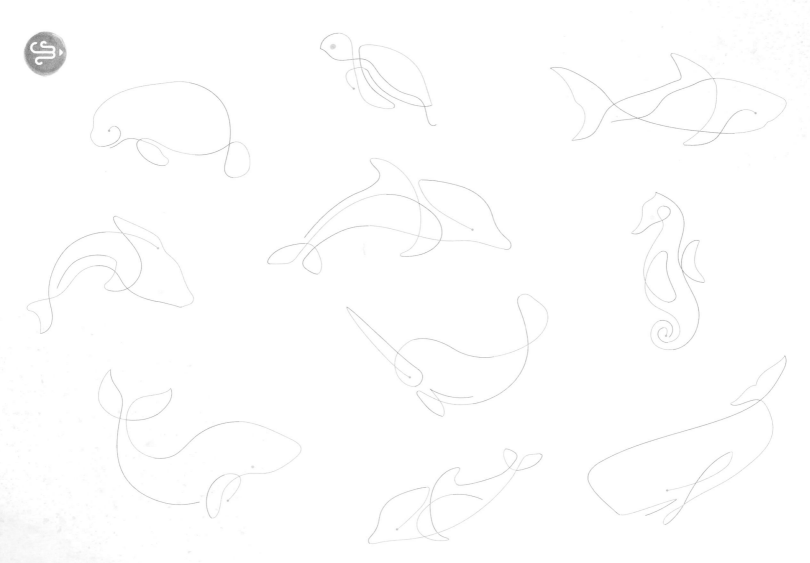

Bring these sea creatures to life with
tranquil, flowing movements.

Open your mind

When we look directly at something, we use the centre of our visual field. This focused area is called our "foveal" vision and only accounts for 5% of our *actual* visual field.[21] The following exercise helps us to explore our peripheral vision, widening our field of perception.

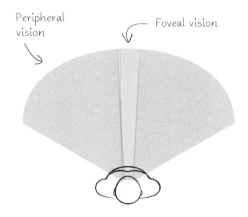

Peripheral vision

Foveal vision

A guided audio "open focus" meditation is available at **drawbreath.com**

What you will achieve here with your visual field can be achieved in all of your other fields of awareness. This widening of attention and awareness can be applied to your hearing, taste and all your internal and external bodily sensations. This is the core skill we develop when learning "open monitoring meditation".

Dr Les Fehmi, a pioneer of biofeedback science, discusses this phenomenon in his book *The Open Focus Brain*. He categorizes four different qualities of focus available to us, each with its own associated physiological state: narrow focus, diffused focus, immersed focus and objective focus. Being in a state of "diffused" focus naturally relaxes the body, while being "immersed" in focus can be intrinsically rewarding. Dr Fehmi believes that many of us rarely leave the state of "narrow" focus – our brains are stuck in problem-solving mode, and as a result our bodies never fully relax.

The purpose of the following exercise is not to draw a perfect representation of the room but to demonstrate, through experience, that our focus is usually limited to a small fraction of our available awareness. But, with minimal conscious effort, we can widen our attention.

Just like the body needs exercise to stay healthy and flexible, so does the mind. Mindfulness is like taking your brain to the gym and giving it a workout.

OPEN YOUR EYES

Choose a place to sit where the shape of the room or the layout of items in the room becomes visually interesting.

Sit comfortably with your book in your lap or on a table in front of you.

Rest your gaze on a place in the room that is a few feet straight ahead of you.

Allow your attention to become focused there. (It may help to place an object in the centre of your gaze to focus on.)

Without moving your gaze, transfer your attention around the room by shifting your awareness to different parts of your visual field. Your eyes should remain focused on the object in front of you throughout.

Avoid the temptation to look down at the book!

Beginning with the object or place you are looking at, draw simple lines to represent the size and shape of the objects in the room and their locations in relation to each other. Use the blank page opposite.

Once you have covered the key objects in the room and the shape of the room, you may wish to add a few details, still keeping your gaze resting in the centre of the room.

Did the change in focus have any effect on your emotional state? Or your body?

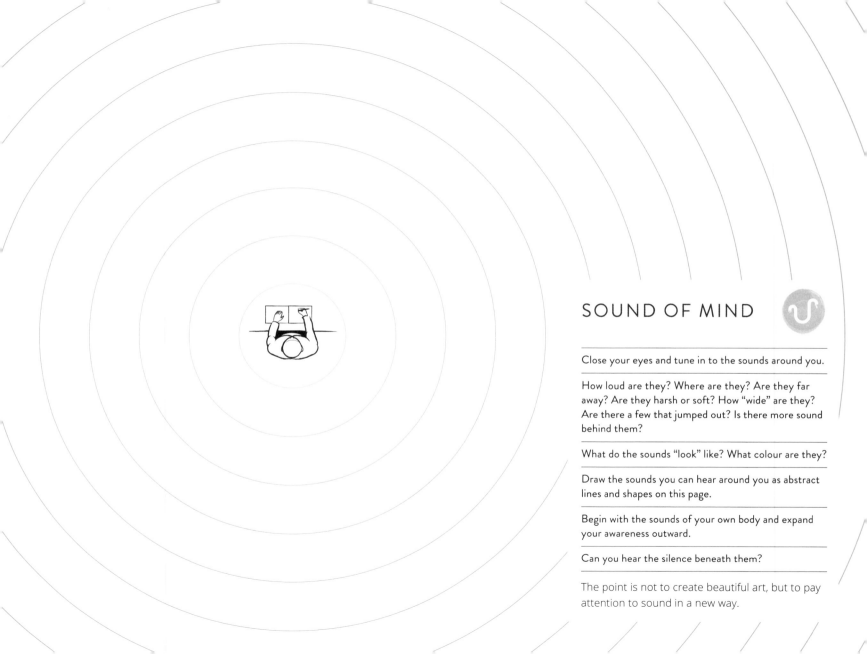

SOUND OF MIND

Close your eyes and tune in to the sounds around you.

How loud are they? Where are they? Are they far away? Are they harsh or soft? How "wide" are they? Are there a few that jumped out? Is there more sound behind them?

What do the sounds "look" like? What colour are they?

Draw the sounds you can hear around you as abstract lines and shapes on this page.

Begin with the sounds of your own body and expand your awareness outward.

Can you hear the silence beneath them?

The point is not to create beautiful art, but to pay attention to sound in a new way.

Coherent thinking

When you breathe rhythmically your internal systems begin to synchronize. Not only do your heart rate, blood pressure and breathing rate become harmonious, the electrical patterns of your brain join in with the symphony.

Rhythmic breathing creates rhythmic brain waves. When these electrical waves are synchronized, connections are more easily made across different areas of the brain. We experience these connections as moments of insight.[22]

This is why we have so many of our most inspired thoughts in the shower or just before we drift off to sleep. These are the moments when our bodies are often most relaxed.

This insight mode in the brain is referred to by its discoverer, Dr Les Fehmi, as "whole brain synchrony" and can be entered into deliberately, through rhythmic breathing exercises.

This means epiphanies are no longer something that you have to wait for. The required brain state can be "hacked into", using breathwork.

TEAR UP THE RULE BOOK

Tear this page down the line on the right to give yourself some notepaper. Notice any feelings of anxiety or exhilaration as you do so. It's unusual to rip out a page from a book.

You are breaking a habit, challenging a preconception about what a book can be, and your body may well register a physical response.

On your newly torn-off sheet, write down some other uses for your pencil. Stop thinking about it as a pencil. What can its new function be? Give yourself one minute to think of as many new uses as you can.

Look away from the page.

Sitting quietly, take ten slow and deep breaths, counting aloud in your head, in for five seconds and out for six.

Now look back at your page.

Did you have any new ideas?

Did any pop into your head unbidden while you were still counting your breath?

NEW USES FOR A PENCIL...

*How you think
is important...*

*... but not how
you think!*

How did you do?

Share your answers –
#DrawBreathBook

Meditation makes you more creative

Even just a few minutes of meditation makes us more inventive in a number of ways, and regular practice has a huge impact on our overall creativity.

By entering a relaxed and receptive state of mind, we become, in a literal sense, more "open-minded" to new ideas and ways of interpreting the world. Our thoughts are subjective, fleeting and often flawed rather than solid, literal interpretations of the world, and seeing them for what they are allows our thinking to become more lateral.

By being present, we are able to "absorb" elements of our environment and our own thoughts more consciously, which, in turn, stores them subconsciously in our short-term working memory. This increases the number of "ingredients" available to us with which we can "cook up" creative solutions. And, by being less distracted by our thoughts, we clear our heads, clearing a path for moments of insight.

By regularly interrupting our patterns of habitual thinking, we naturally become more divergent in our intelligence.

When we tune our awareness to our physical bodies, we are more in touch with our gut feelings and what our hearts are telling us. This offers the artist within each of us new interpretations of the world and deepens our intuition.

By removing the ego from the creative process, we become less protective of our ideas and the things we create. This allows us to detach from them, observe them objectively and improve them accordingly. In other words, they begin to have a life of their own and grow more organically. Our role becomes that of the gardener growing flowers, nurturing them, enjoying their aromas and the company of the birds and other wildlife that they feed.

Creativity can be created

True creativity rarely feels like a conscious process. When faced with a problem, we often scratch our heads, chew our pencils and try to think of a solution... to no avail. Then, later on, when we've moved on to something else... Bam! The idea shoots out of our subconscious and hits us squarely between the eyes. We congratulate ourselves on our ingenuity, but are we truly responsible for these moments of inspiration? Our experience suggests not.

The poets and artists of ancient Greece believed inspiration to come from divine sources, fortuitous interference from the Muses. A gift from the Gods. The word "inspiration" comes from the Latin *"inspirare"*, meaning literally, "breathe into". As though the Gods are blowing onto the embers of our minds and fanning the flames.

Wherever ideas might come from, creative thinking is important for much more than just... well... being "creative".

Creativity is a skill. A form of problem solving where we take two or more different ideas and combine them in a novel way to make something original.

It doesn't just apply to art and design, where the goal itself is to create something new. Creative thinking is needed for all of life's problems, from the mundane organization of our daily timetable or writing emails, to setting authentic life goals and getting the most out of our personal relationships.

The more creative we become, the more adaptable and flexible we can be, and the more resilient we are to life's challenges.

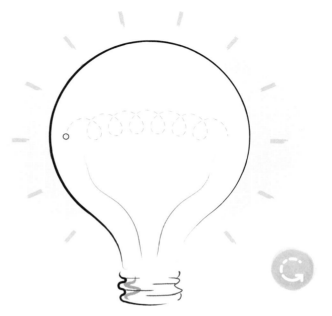

NOVELTY LEADS TO NOVEL IDEAS

Routine is useful; it's convenient, it's comfortable and it saves time. Having a plan stops us from endlessly dithering so that we can get the most out of our days. But on a larger scale, it can speed up psychological time. When we are young everything is new and summers seem to last forever. But as we age, we get into routines and we stop having as many new experiences. The years start to go by faster... When we rely on routine, we stop exploring. We escape the challenging nature of new experiences, but as a result we don't need to experiment, think or create new memories. Our creative faculties wither like an unused muscle. The antidote is to make a routine out of seeking new experiences, breaking habits and challenging yourself to find new ways of doing things.

Draw the guided practice above with the opposite hand to the one you would naturally use.

If you are right-handed, draw with your left hand and vice versa.

How did it feel? Could you feel your brain and body working together in new ways?

ACKNOWLEDGING THE NEGATIVE

Meditation isn't about training ourselves to focus on the positive so that we can ignore the negative. Often, it is the very suppression of negative thoughts that causes our anxiety. It is our resistance to pain that causes suffering.

Draw this cloud in time with the constant movement of your breath.

Allowing negative thoughts to enter our minds, rather than repressing them, helps us to see them for what they are; ephemeral, fleeting mental events. They move through the mind's eye like clouds in the sky. They are impermanent.

By acknowledging pain and exploring it with curiosity and compassion, we can change our relationship to it. If you have a niggling pain in your body now, rather than trying to wish it away, try to go deeply into it, try to pinpoint its exact location, and actually try to feel it *more* intensely.

What shape is the pain in three-dimensional space? Try to visualize it within your body.

The harder you search for the location of the pain, the harder it is to pinpoint. You will notice it is always changing, always in flow.

The pain may even dissolve slightly. Fear of the pain adds another layer of suffering. The same is true for our fear of negative thoughts.

SEEKING OUT THE POSITIVE

As human beings we have evolved to have a natural tendency toward negativity. This "negativity bias" is a useful evolutionary adaptation. It's a more effective survival strategy to mistakenly see a rock in the distance as a sabre-toothed tiger than it is to see a sabre-toothed tiger as a rock. Our ancestors kept their guard up, survived and passed their pessimistic genes onto us. The optimistic cavemen sat down on rocks that jumped up and ate them. And their happy-go-lucky genes were lost forever.

Just as we can train our minds to focus on our experience as well as our thoughts, we can train ourselves to naturally seek out the positive, rather than the negative.

Take a stroll around your house and look for things that are aesthetically beautiful, emotionally resonant or just naturally give you positive feelings you can't explain.

Make a collage on this page with doodles of these things that you walk by every day. How often do you notice them?

Take your time on this task, spend perhaps thirty minutes seeking, drawing, moving, seeking, drawing, moving.

Aim to fill the page with at least 15 distinct doodles.

Entering this upbeat seeking mode will have an effect on how you see the world for a short time after the exercise. Doing it regularly will have a more lasting effect.

The quality of your drawings is not important. It is the seeking and exploring element of this task that makes a difference.

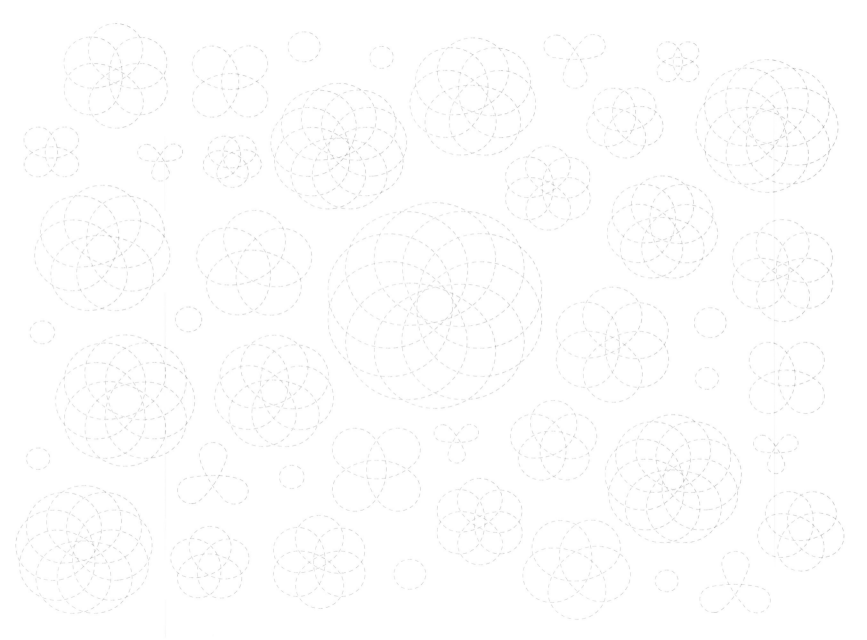

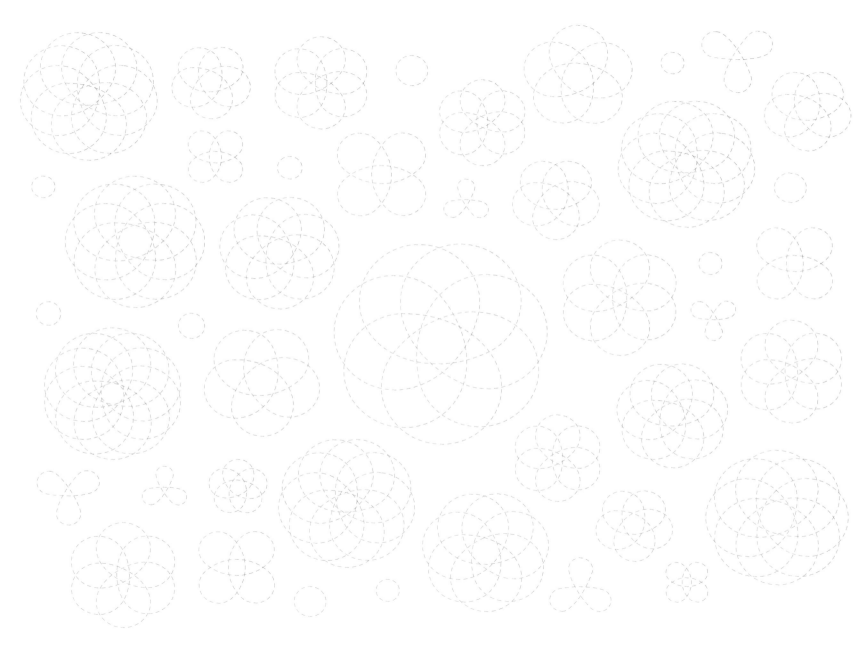

Remember to observe a few natural breaths before and after each doodling exercise.

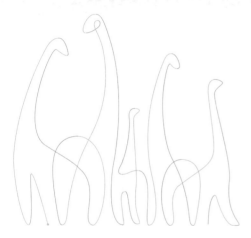

Deep in our evolutionary past, our amygdala kept us safe from predators by kick-starting our fight-or-flight response... but now it can make us panic about things that really aren't that life threatening, like deadlines, or what shoes to wear!

Help this family of brachiosaurus to stay calm and on the lookout with nice, long breaths.

"Monkey mind" is an ancient Buddhist term that describes the mind in its restless state, jumping from one thought to the next with indecision and anxiety.

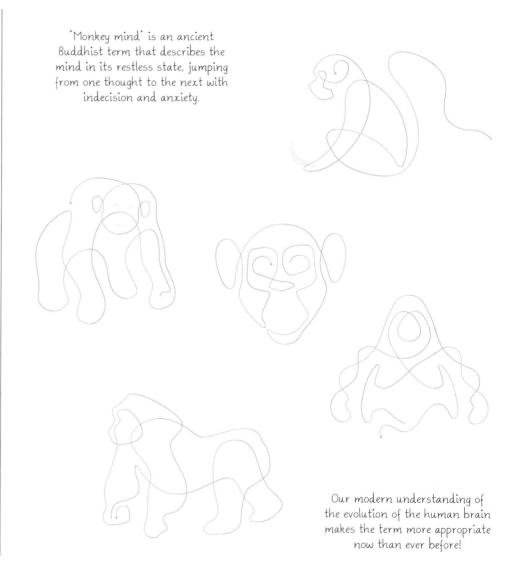

Our modern understanding of the evolution of the human brain makes the term more appropriate now than ever before!

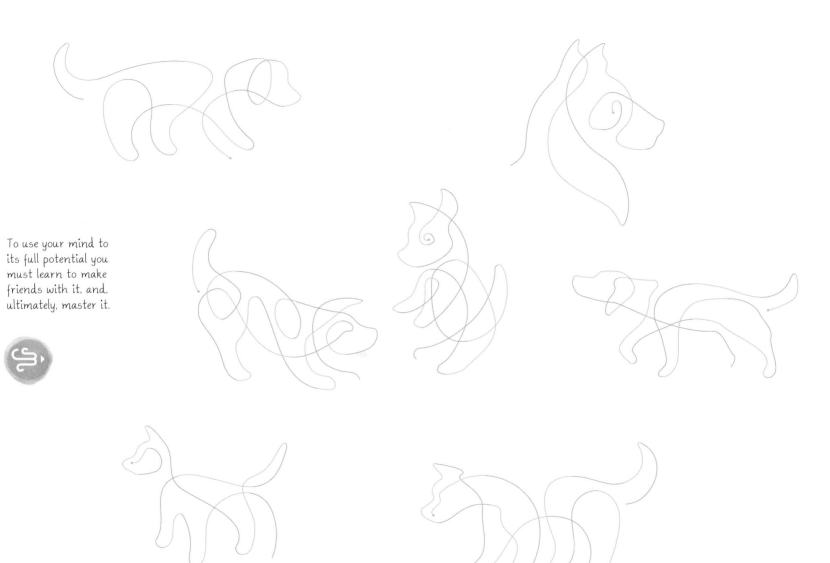

To use your mind to its full potential you must learn to make friends with it, and, ultimately, master it.

OPEN LINES OF COMMUNICATION

When we focus on our breathing, we calm our minds and our new perspective on thoughts means we are less likely to be drawn into reactive behaviour. The activation of our PNS means we are more capable of releasing oxytocin – the "love hormone".

The parts of our brain that are associated with empathy become more active and we get better at understanding other people.

We become better communicators and our relationships can improve as a result.

Using lines drawn with mindful observation of the breath, make a clear connection between these telegraph poles and create an open line of communication.

As you do so, notice what is unique about each inhalation and exhalation.

Drawing the path of the breath offers a constant for our awareness – a focal point for each second as it merges with the next. Each point in time is noticed and recorded as it slips into part of the fluid whole we call our experience.

The pencil touching the page is an anchor that keeps you here and now. The image becomes a representation of your internal experience in the external world. A flowing record of the present moment as it evolves.

Laughter is contagious

We are thirty times more likely to laugh if we are around other people... It's as though company makes jokes thirty times funnier![23]

Yawning, laughing, crying. These are all just strange and often involuntary forms of breathing, and they are all contagious! They are also highly social, communicating how we feel.

These aren't the only breathing patterns we can pass on to other people; they are just the most noticeable, visually and audibly.

Breathing patterns were used as a form of communication long before we evolved the capacity for speech. Mirror neurons in your brain notice the breathing patterns of the people around you and give you a taste of the corresponding emotion so that you know how they feel. You converge emotionally. What emotions are you sending out into the world?

By breathing calmly, you can subconsciously affect the people around you with your breathing pattern and, in doing so, change their mental state from stressed to calm. If you have children or pets, see if you can pass your breathing pattern on to them. You may be surprised by how easy it is!

LAUGHTER LINES

Use your breath to transmit the positive mental state from the first person all the way to the last.

Take this thought with you when you leave the house and see if you can pass on your calm breathing pattern to anyone else.

Yawning is an ancient signal that we are relaxed and comfortable in another's presence. Stop stifling your yawns and tell your friends to take it as a compliment!

Ride your next few breaths and let the spontaneous flow direct you as you chart the path of this sky-writing plane — include a few loop-the-loops!

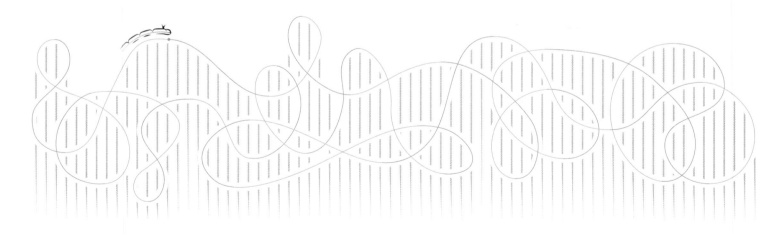

Tracing breath-drawings with the tip of your finger can be just as interesting as drawing with a pencil — give it a go on this rollercoaster.

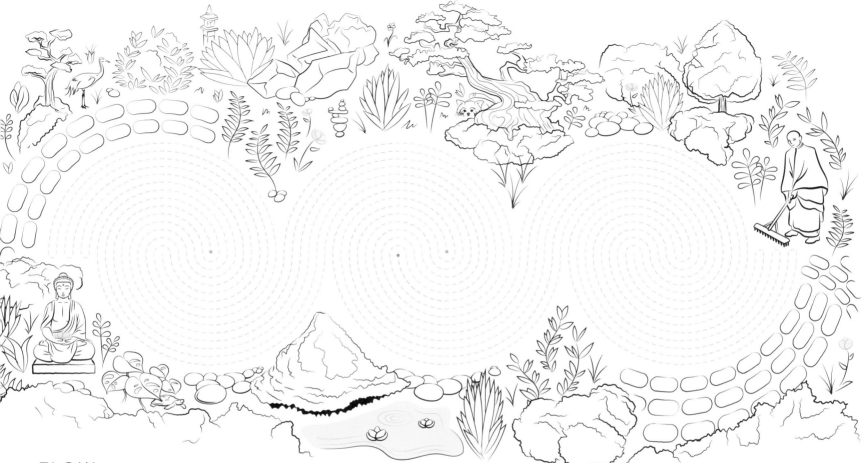

FLOW

When a task is challenging but achievable, we can completely lose ourselves in it – we enter a state of naturally intense, intrinsically rewarding focus. When we are "in the zone" on a project, we become absorbed in it, while simultaneously enjoying the feeling of immersion and calm concentration. We lose our sense of time. We lose ourselves in flow.

Help this monk rake his sand garden into a beautiful pattern and achieve a state of peaceful, flowing concentration.

This illustration has three starting points and will take a while to complete... so feel free to complete it in three separate sessions.

Mindlessness

We've focused a lot so far on mindful states, but what about the benefits of mindless activities? Mindfulness is only one type of focus that we are usually lacking, but what of other focusing styles?

Were you ever told off in school for doodling on your exercise book when you were supposed to be listening? Recent studies suggest that doodling isn't a sign of distraction. In fact, doodling while listening to new information allows your brain to concentrate, in a diffused way, for longer periods of time and retain more information.

One study showed that short-term memory retention among doodlers improved by 29% when compared to a control group.[24] Normally, when we multitask, we see the opposite result; our focusing capacity is halved as it splits itself between two inputs. But doodling not only improves focus, it also relieves stress, helping us to relax, which allows us to be more creative with the new information.

ONE LINER

Without lifting your pencil from the paper, draw a one-line doodle.

Let the pencil make its own journey across the page.

Allow each movement to correspond with the spontaneous shape of its own wake.

Enjoy the experience of not having a plan for the simple image you are making.

Without a goal in mind, keep adding to your doodle, allowing it to evolve and take shape.

"Drawing takes time, a line has time in it."

– David Hockney

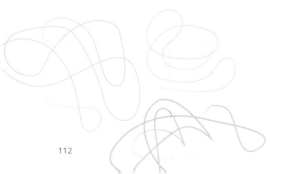

DOODLE FOR YOUR NOODLE

Some psychologists believe that when we doodle in a free-form way, we are allowing elements of our subconscious to express themselves and come to the surface.[25] This helps us to be in touch with, organize and reconcile important elements of our psyche that we are barely aware of.

Doodle on this page one mark at a time.

Draw the first line with your dominant hand and the next with your other hand, and continue switching between hands, line after line.

Use a different colour for each hand.

Let each new mark be a response to the last and a part of the whole.

Take your time and allow the resultant drawing to be an abstract visual "conversation" between the two hemispheres of your brain.

You are not trying to draw anything in particular. Just allow your pencil to flow across the page.

Let each line take about one exhalation to complete and think about your next line as you inhale.

Draw. Pause. Consider. And repeat.

Give yourself time to complete your drawing.

CSI

You only ever draw three types of line: C shapes, S shapes and I shapes. Thinking of your lines as these simple, distinctive elements compels you to draw one line at a time.

Although this is a simple insight, it was a complete revelation to me. It changed how I draw.

LUCKY STARS

Join the dots on this page at random to create new constellations.

Allow each penstroke to take one breath to complete.

Do any images present themselves?

Name your new constellations.

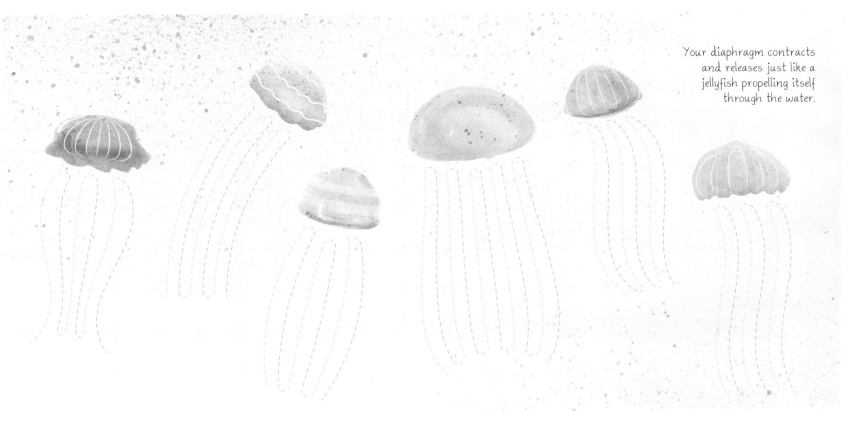

Your diaphragm contracts and releases just like a jellyfish propelling itself through the water.

SPINELESS, BRAINLESS, FLAWLESS

Jellyfish have it easy. They don't have a prefrontal lobe. They don't worry about where they have been or where they're going. They use their bodies to gently propel themselves through the water on their migration, but they also surrender to the current of the ocean. They do not fight it, they use the natural flow of their environment as it changes from one moment to the next.

Use your breath to draw the tentacles on this shoal of jellyfish and help them move with the flow.

As much as you can, allow the breath to happen naturally and report your observations to the page.

Another wei

We don't always have to do things to get things done. Just as we can actively inhale but exhale passively with no effort, in non-doing, by subtly shifting our point of view and observing ourselves in action, we are able to ride life's flow more organically and without strain. This concept is called "Wu Wei" in Chinese Taoism. Sometimes simply **being** is as important as **doing** for our productivity and happiness.

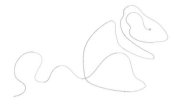

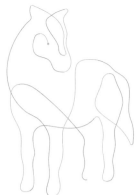

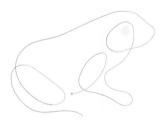

Spending time outdoors in nature isn't just good for you physically, it's good for you mentally too. In Japan the pastime is fondly called "forest bathing".

Go outside and find a nice, peaceful place to sit. Use some "fresh air" to draw these animals of the forest in time with your breath.

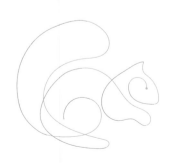

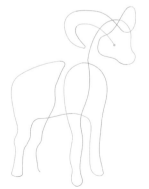

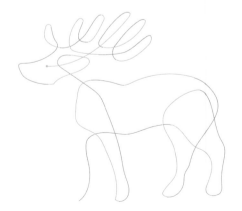

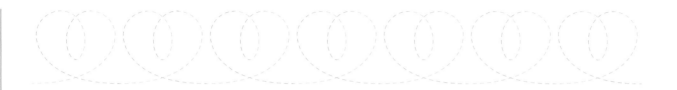

You are not what you think

In the first part of the book we learned how the breath can help us to harness our energy, boost our vitality and support us in feeling grounded within our bodies.

In this section we have studied how, although we identify with our thoughts most of the time, we are not our thoughts – they are just optional ways of viewing and interpreting the world. Used creatively, they are ways of learning from our past or planning for the future.

"He who knows himself is enlightened."

– Lao Tzu

So, if we are not our thoughts... what are we?

The final part of the book explores how the mind, body and breath are one. And, by shifting our perspective with drawing techniques, we will see how deeply connected we are to the world, the universe and the people around us.

If you feel there's a
piece of you missing...

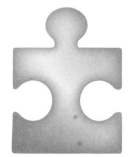

... it's probably
your inner peace

PART 3

SPIRIT

Prana
Yogic tradition

Perhaps the oldest known breath philosophy, "prana" is the fundamental energy that makes up everything that exists in the world, and it's in a constant state of flow. The word also means "breath" in Sanskrit. "Pranayama" is the system of breath control in yoga; for millennia yogic practitioners have used breathing techniques to balance, focus and increase the flow of prana through their bodies and minds. Although the idea of yoga often conjures images of acrobatic contortionists in impossible positions, the yogic postures are secondary to breathing practices, and are primarily designed to create a state of healthy prana flow or vitality in the body.

Qi
Chinese medicine

Pronounced and sometimes spelled "chi", as in **qi**gong and tai **chi**, the qi concept is fundamental to Chinese medicine and martial arts. These ancient philosophies teach that we are all manifestations of qi energy. Qigong practitioners heal and strengthen their bodies and empower their minds using breathing and visualization techniques to control and improve the flow of their qi. Some historians believe that the ideas of qi and prana may have shared roots dating back thousands of years. Qi and prana can both be understood as our inner feelings of energy and vitality; you know when it is lacking, because it's harder to get out of bed!

Ki
Japanese culture

When the concept of qi was taken from China to Japan in the sixth century, it became an enduring element of Japanese philosophy. It forms a fundamental part of Japanese ideas about inspiration and subtle energy systems. It is also the basis for modern Japanese martial arts such as ai**ki**do, which teaches practitioners to harness their energy flow through visualization and breathing techniques. The goal in aikido is to defeat your opponent without causing them harm.

Breath of life

Many spiritual and medicinal traditions around the world equate the breath with our life-force, energy or spirit.

Lung
Tibetan Buddhism

Not to be confused with the organs we use to breathe! In Tibetan Buddhism "lung" translates as "breath" or "wind" and forms an idea similar to yogic prana. Tsa lung is a Tibetan practice which shares a lot of its philosophy and techniques with yoga, and is used to balance the body internally and expand the mind. "Tsa" means "space", "vessel" or "channel". Tsa lung literally translates as "channelling wind".

"Light" these candles with your breath after reading each paragraph.

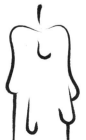

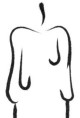

Psyche
Greek philosophy

Psyche, a Greek word that we now use to mean "mind" (the origin of our word "psychology"), originally meant "breath", "life" or "soul". The Greeks also referred to the concept of *"pneuma"*, our life force or "breath of life"; an important mystery to the first Western philosophers and analogous to our modern Western idea of the "soul".

Spirit
Western Christianity

The word spirit, as in "Holy Spirit", has its roots in the Latin word *"spiritus"*, meaning breath. In the West, we associate the words "spirit" and "soul" with the idea of an animating life force; something invisible and eternal that exists inside our physical bodies and gives them life... but that is made of something altogether different from them. In the story of Genesis, God "breathes life" into Adam.

Ruach
Judaism

In Hebrew "ruach" is a similar concept to "spirit" in Christianity but it still shares its meaning with the words "breath" and "air" in modern Hebrew. It forms a base for many of the Judaic names for God, such as "Ruach HaKodesh" or "Ruach Elohim", which translate roughly as "Spirit of God" or "Divine Breath". In the Torah and the Old Testament, God is often referred to as manifesting and interacting with humans in the form of wind.

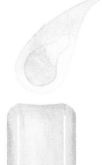

Even our Western scientific words have their origins in these ancient ideas. "Respiration" from the Latin *"spiritus"*, meaning "breath", shares its root meaning with our idea of "spirit" as an animating force.

Breathing is undeniably more than the transmission of air. It is the conversion of energy from the physical world into consciousness; it animates us. It affects our whole being on a physical, experiential, emotional and energetic level.

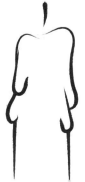

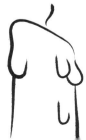

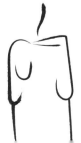

The internal arts

Esoteric Eastern concepts about life-force energy that can be felt in the body and strengthened or manipulated through the breath (for all kinds of incredible health benefits) sit neatly alongside a corresponding Western idea we discussed earlier, that of "interoception".

Interoceptive ability is directly parallel to these ideas. When our PNS is active and our inner sensory channels become clearer during deep rhythmic breathing, we become more aware of our inner world. Our internal channels of perception "switch on" through the vagus nerve. The more our interoception improves, the better our bodies are at balancing homoeostasis... and the healthier we become.

The combined internal sensations of blood flow and oxygen levels is our body monitoring its own energy levels and homeostatic equilibrium; we experience these feelings as an overlapping, vibrating, energy-like quality.

Without anything visible to create a frame of reference, "energy" and "life force" feel like appropriate descriptions of these sensations.

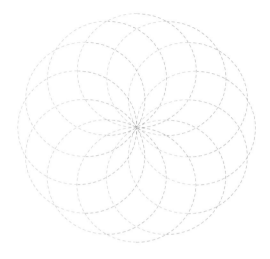

Since the respiratory system *is* our energy system and ergo our life force, these terms are appropriate scientifically speaking as well. With these observations in mind, the ideas of qi and prana feel less like esoteric "new age" concepts and more like fundamental, important and widely ignored parts of our dialogue about the human experience that Western science, medicine and culture as a whole are currently lacking.

In qigong and yoga, visualization techniques are used to strengthen qi or prana. If you are uncomfortable with these terms, please read "interoception" in their place as we move onto these visualization practices.

Qigong ond tai chi are sometimes referred to as "the internal arts".

We simply don't have a corresponding system of creative visualization and movement in the West to channel and improve our interoception in time with the breath.

This is why yoga and mindfulness have become so popular so quickly. They fulfil a desperate need!

Complete these mandalas one breath at a time, using the circle technique we learned on page 40.

Visualize the oxygen flooding in and energizing your body on your inhalation, and imagine you are expelling negative energy with each exhalation.

How does this affect your inner feelings?

Do you have more energy? Or a different kind of energy?

This geometric "fruit of life" design consists of 61 interlocking circles. That's 61 breaths. It will take a while to complete... so take your time!

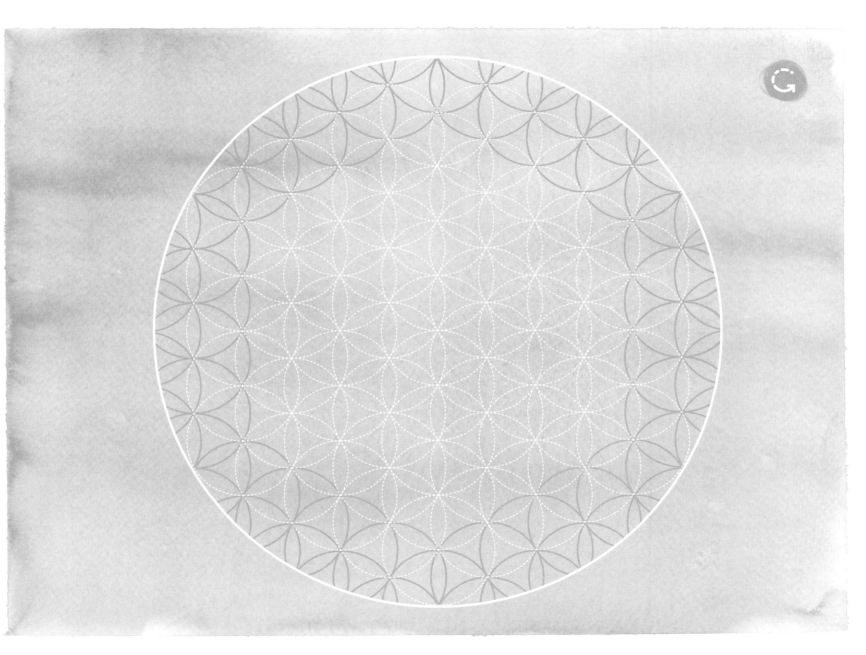

CIRCLES OF LIFE

Ancient traditional visualization techniques span across countries and cultures. Chinese qigong, Indian yoga and Russian martial arts all share variations on the technique of visualizing the breath as energy flowing through the body.

The yogic chakras are energy centres located along the midline of the body that spin like wheels.

For thousands of years the yogis have believed we can "activate" these chakras through breathing and visualization techniques.

This ancient system, grounded in subjective experience, corresponds with modern science's account of how we can activate the perceptions of our inner body by stimulating the vagus nerve with deep and rhythmic breathing.

Starting at the base, breathe "into" and "out of" each of the chakras in turn.

Visualize the breath moving the wheel of your chakra like a water mill.

Draw using the colour traditionally associated with each chakra as you turn the wheel with your breath (indicated opposite).

Go around each circle three times using three breath cycles.

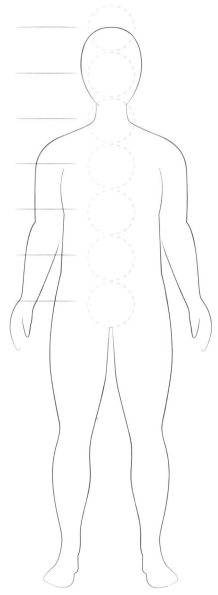

Crown: Violet

Third eye: Indigo

Throat: Blue

Heart: Green

Solar plexus: Yellow

Sacral: Orange

Root: Red

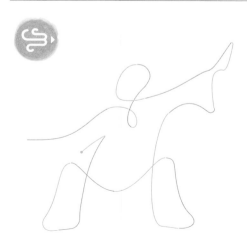

BREATH MOVING

Qigong practitioners use a technique called "breath moving" where they imagine breathing into and out of different parts of their bodies for different benefits.

As you trace this breath-drawing, imagine your breath flowing around your body along the path that the pencil is taking around the figure.

Visualize each breath oxygenating and renewing the part of your body wherever the pencil is tracing.

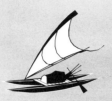

THE DIVINE BREATH

The Polynesian word for breath is *"ha"*. It also translates as "the divine breath of life". It's a beautifully onomatopoeic word that forms the foundation of their salutary blessings and thanks: *"alo**ha**"*, *"ma**ha**lo"*.

When Captain Cook's crew members first sailed to Polynesia and asked where they had arrived, the locals replied "**Ha**waii", meaning "We reside in the breath of the divine." To the advanced seafaring peoples of the Pacific, the breath, the wind and the world are one.

When the Western sailors refused the traditional Polynesian greeting of touching noses to share breath, they forever became known as "**Ha**oles" – "those who do not breathe".

Help these Polynesian sailors on their journey!

Use your breath to draw their wake and give this image movement as they voyage across the sea to find new islands. Imagine your exhalation filling their sails.

Passively observe your automatic breathing pattern as though the universe is breathing you.

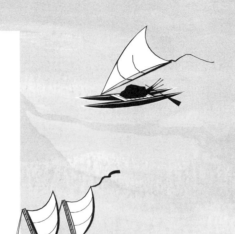

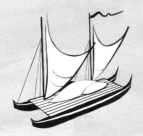

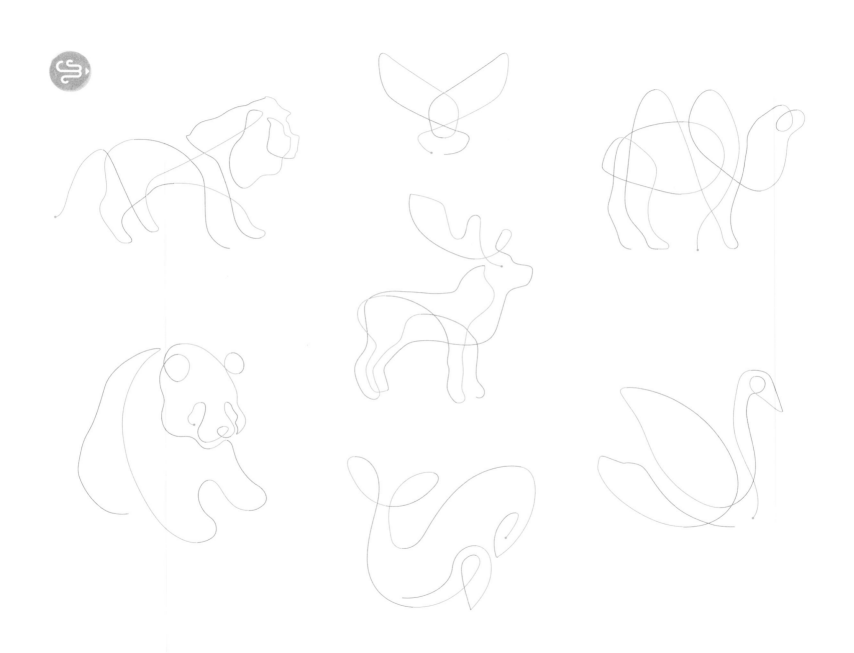

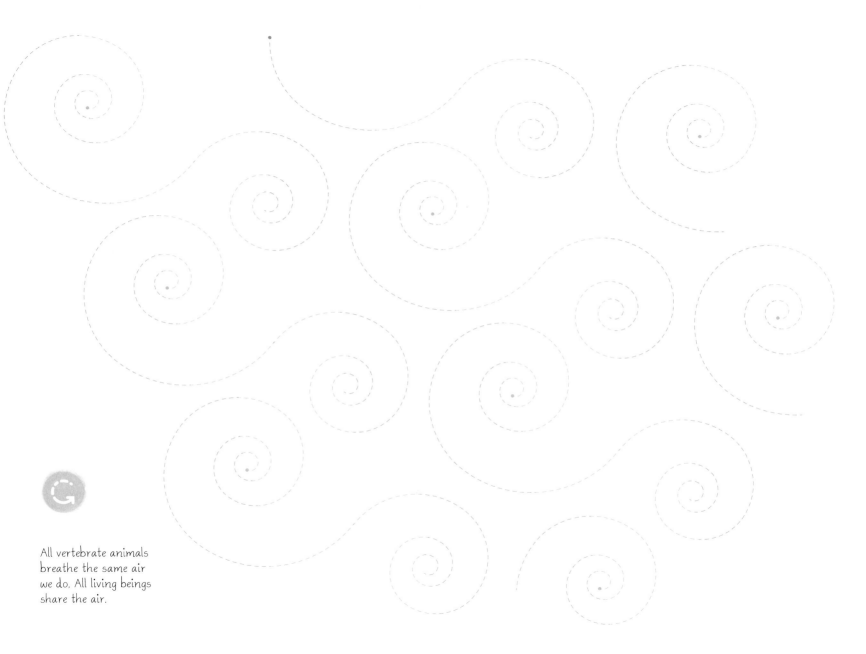

All vertebrate animals
breathe the same air
we do, All living beings
share the air.

The cuddle hormone

Through simple breathing exercises it's possible to change our blood chemistry and increase our ability to love and feel connected to other people and the world at large.

When our PNS is active, we feel more relaxed, our focus broadens and our bodies release oxytocin into the bloodstream more readily. Oxytocin, sometimes called the "cuddle" or "love" hormone, increases our feelings of connectedness to the people around us.

When oxytocin is present in the bloodstream, our capacity for empathy is elevated – our ability to understand other people on an emotional level improves.

When the SNS is active, it is difficult for the body to release and feel the effects of oxytocin.

Not only does the presence of oxytocin increase our capacity for moments of love and connection; moments of love and connection increase the sensitivity of our vagus nerve.[26]

A traditional guided audio "loving kindness" meditation is available at drawbreath.com

"Love is the bridge between you and everything."

~ Rumi

WARM-HEARTED

Think of someone you love or care about and hold their face or name in your mind while you draw a heart on the page opposite.

Make the heart about the size of your thumbnail.

On your next inhalation, visualize warm energy flowing in through your nose and down into your heart. Feel the energy filling your heart, overflowing down your arm, out of your pen and onto the page as you colour in the heart.

As you colour the heart and fill it with this energy, imagine the positive energy filling the person you have chosen.

Keep breathing into your heart and feeling the energy flowing from your breath to your heart, to the page, until the heart is coloured in.

Do this once for someone you love, once for someone you feel indifferent to (perhaps a stranger you recently interacted with) and once for someone you feel negatively toward.

If you find it difficult to think of someone in your personal life who you are willing to do this for, select someone from popular culture instead... Perhaps a politician!

Feel free to include any animals you know as well as people in this "loving kindness" meditation.

How does your heart feel after doing this exercise?

Keep coming back to this page and repeating this practice until it is filled with compassionate hearts.

We are all one.

(But at least we have each other for company!)

Slow, deep breathing activates the PNS, allowing us to release oxytocin and helping us to feel more connected to the people around us.

Deep breathing stops you being shallow

Use a single line to help this family of elephants stay connected trunk to tail.

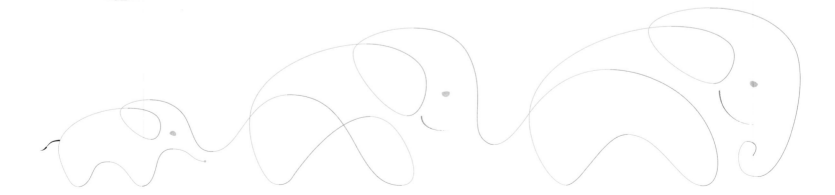

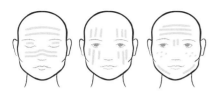

INVISIBLE WAR PAINT

Clap your hands once, and without separating them, rub them together until you generate heat.

Very slowly begin to move them apart, feeling the heat of each hand radiating into the other.

Continue separating them slowly and notice any energetic feelings in your palms.

Gently use the sensations of energy in your hands to "paint" a symmetrical pattern onto your face by softly stroking or tapping your cheekbones, forehead and jawline.

Notice if this releases any tension in your face.

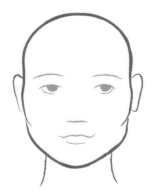
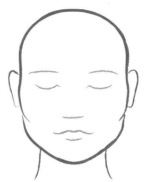
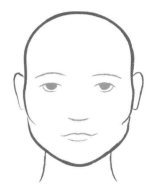

Deep in our evolutionary past when we were primates living in large groups, grooming would have been a daily social experience. For millions of years the act of grooming was foundational to group unity and individual feelings of self-worth. Gentle sensations of touch activate the PNS and release oxytocin to prepare the body and mind for a bonding experience.

In caressing your face like this you have just engaged in self compassion and subtly changed your physiology and mental state.

How often are you kind to yourself like this?

Repeat the exercise, experimenting with what feels good and use your findings to design some unique "war paint" for yourself on the templates above.

Use your "invisible war paint" as a ritual to prepare yourself the next time you are facing a stressful situation.

This can also be a soothing exercise to help prepare you for sleep.

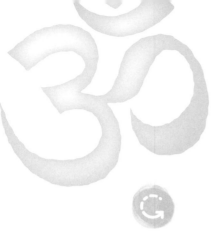

OM

In Hindu spirituality, OM represents everything, from the universe to the soul. It is the cosmic sound, "the sound of the universe".

To some Hindus the sound of OM symbolizes the breath of the creator God Brahma creating reality – exhaling the entire universe and everything in it into existence. It denotes everything that is and simultaneously acknowledges its impermanence – an exhalation precedes an inhalation.

Make the "OM" sound as you complete the descenders on this guided practice. Lengthen the sound for as long as you can.

It will help to break it into three sounds. Start with your mouth open, then purse your lips before closing your mouth completely – "ah-oo-mm".

Use the sound to create natural resistance and vibration, lengthening the exhalation and enjoying the vibrations through your body.

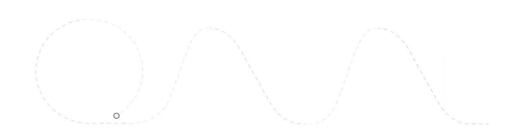

A study in 2011 used fMRI imaging to research the impact of OM breathing on the brain. The participants who chanted "OM" while in the fMRI scanners displayed much lower activation states in their amygdala. The results were comparable to the effects of vagal nerve stimulation, suggesting that the combination of vibration and resistance in OM breathing "switches off" ancient parts of our brains associated with fight-or-flight, allowing for higher states of consciousness.[27]

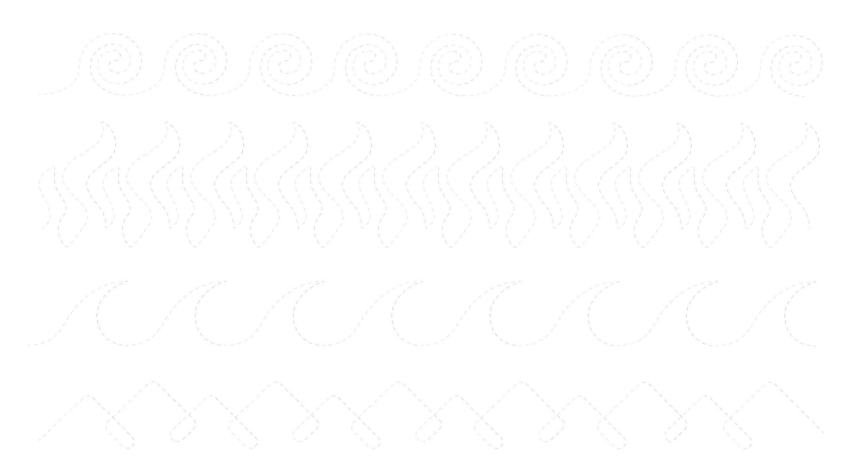

 Since the dawn of humanity we have contemplated what the world is made of. In ancient times people believed that everything was made of four elements in different combinations – earth, wind, fire and water.

Today, we describe the world in terms of atoms and forces. Whatever the labels we give to matter, everything in the universe is fundamentally made out of one thing: energy, vibrating and oscillating at different wavelengths.

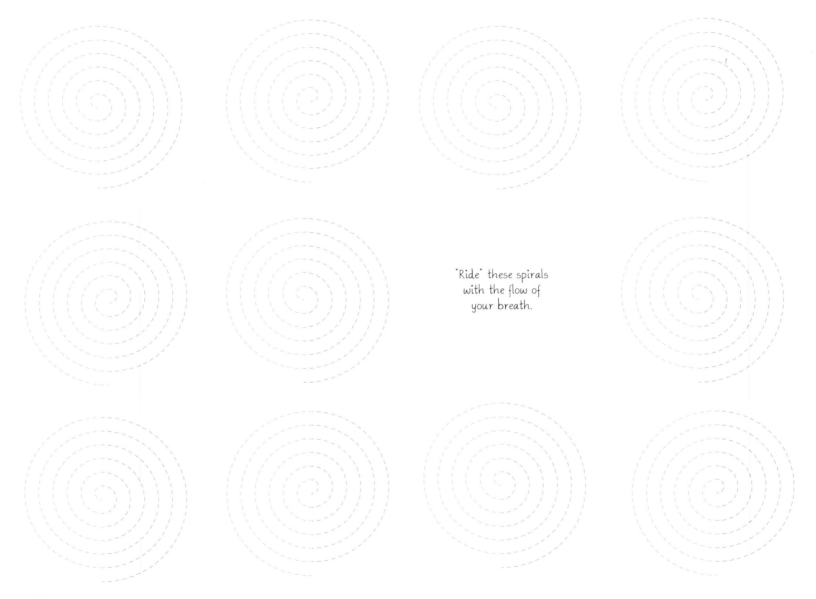

"Ride" these spirals
with the flow of
your breath.

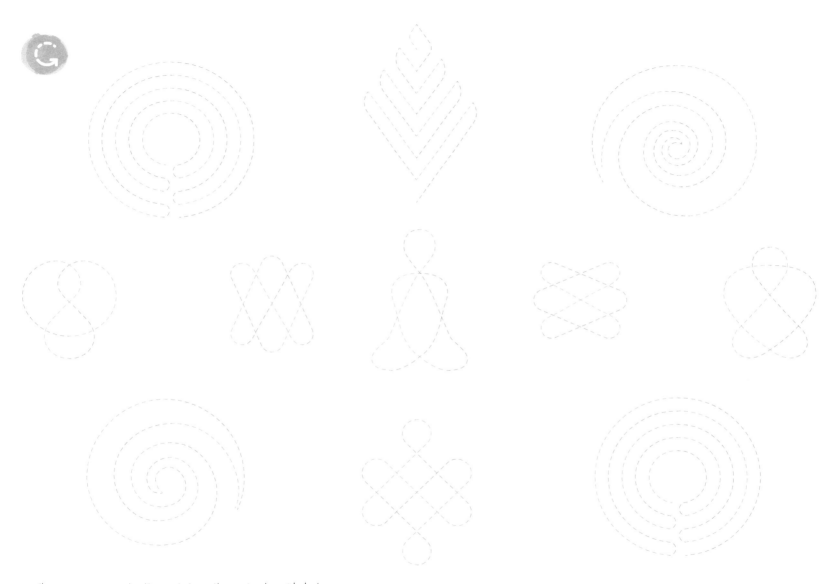

Choose your own starting point on these simple guided shapes.

"Everyone can draw.
Far from being a rare
gift, only possessed by
the "artists" among us,
drawing can be as natural
and instinctive to us as
breathing – if we let it."

– Wendy Ann Greenhalgh

Art of the state

When learning to draw, we learn to truly see. Often, when someone finds drawing difficult, it is because they are not drawing what they are *seeing with their eye*, they are drawing what they are *projecting with their mind*.

If you place a house plant in front of a novice artist and ask them to draw it, they will draw you a house plant. It will be a drawing of *a* house plant, but it won't be the one that's in front of them. It will have leaves and a stem, perhaps some flowers and a pot. These elements may be in an arrangement roughly similar to how they appear on the subject, but that's where the similarities will end.

In her influential 1979 book *Drawing on the Right Side of the Brain*, artist and author Betty Edwards describes two modes of seeing the world that correspond to the functions of our different brain hemispheres. In simple terms, the left side of the brain is verbal and analytical, the right side is visual and emotional. The left side is for methodical problem solving, while its counterpart is for intuitive response.

The right hemisphere sees the world, the left labels and categorizes it, weaving it into a simplified story it can understand.

(These distinctions should not be confused with the qualities specific to the insula that we discussed on page 74.)

When our eyes look at the plant, our mind simplifies it. It's seen plants before, it doesn't have time to study every plant in detail; the left brain labels it "plant" and moves on. Even under further consideration, the infinitesimally complex elements that make up the plant are abridged: "leaves", "flowers", "pot".

When we draw for the first time, these mental labels are all we can see. They are in the way. We draw the labels we are "hearing" in our mind and the symbols we are projecting onto the world. Rather than the individual lines, shades and textures that we are seeing with our eyes, we draw the concept of a plant through a collage of crude and simplified symbols. We draw the words in our mind rather than the shapes in front of us.

This drawing example is a microcosm of our experience in general. We experience the world through the eyes of our dominant, verbal, thinking state of mind; our "left" brain. Instead of experiencing the world directly, we simplify it, dividing it up in our minds and seeing only the rudimentary symbols we project onto our reality.

When you're right, you're right

According to Edwards, learning to draw from life requires a mental shift from "left" to "right" – from verbal to visual – from labelling to observing. Rather than seeing the labels we give to things, we can learn to see the things themselves.

In this sense, drawing from life is a shortcut to a mindful state. It's a way of moving from abstract judgement to direct experience. Not just a rewarding hobby, drawing helps us to practise changing our modes of perception at will.

How do we achieve this shift in perspective? How do we stop judging and start observing?

The exercises on the following pages explore ways of "switching off" the verbal mind, and letting the visual mind take over.

Even if you think you can't draw, have a go at the tasks on the next few pages and you may be surprised at just how accurate you can be. The process of committedly seeing things as they are trains us to notice our immediate judgements and see past them to the object of our awareness as it truly is.

You may be surprised by how accurate you can be, even if you have never really felt confident drawing before.

Now, starting in the bottom right and drawing one line at a time, copy the image that's in the blue box into the pink box.

FLIPPIN' GOOD DRAWING

When we draw things upside down, our verbal mind gives up on trying to figure out what's in front of it and "switches off", allowing the visual mind to take over. In this state we find it easier to stop labelling and draw what we actually see.

First, turn the book 180 degrees so that the image opposite is upside down.

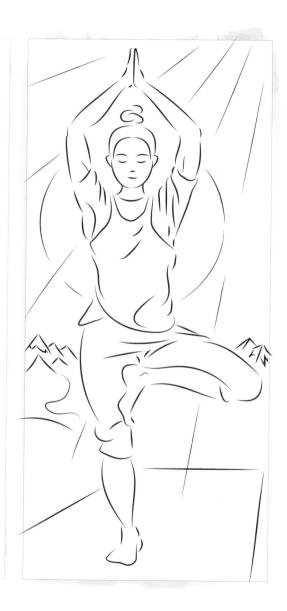

GRID UNLOCK

By dividing an image into smaller parts with a grid system and focusing on a single box, we no longer see the image in the same way. We stop seeing the concept of the thing "as a whole", and start seeing the minute details as they are... as lines and shapes that can be easily copied.

Drawing just one section at a time, copy this image into the grid below.

Avoid the temptation to carry your pen over the grid line until you have finished the box you are working on – take your time.

As you draw, notice the tendency of the verbal mind to "butt in" with value judgements about your work. Whether positive or negative, this is the ego attempting to protect itself from looking foolish. It is fear. Observe your inner critic, let the thoughts come and go and enjoy the process. Nobody is marking your work.

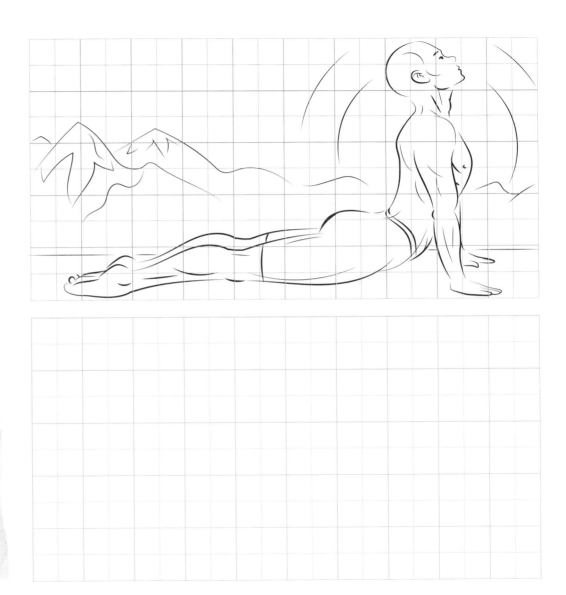

HANDY TIPS

Draw around the outline of your hand onto this grid.

Copy the resulting drawing into the grid on the opposite page.

If you can look at the contents of your own mind with the same non-judgemental curiosity with which you observe the subjects of your drawing, how will your mental life be different?

Don't just copy the shape of the hand – copy all of the imperfections, all of the unintentional wobbles and breaks you created while tracing your hand.

Remember, you are not drawing your hand, you are drawing the line on the page that represents your hand.

LOOK!

If you watch someone drawing from life, you will notice they spend most of the time looking down at their sketchbook. They take a few furtive glances up toward their subject and then look back down at the page. This is backward. As soon as you look down, you are drawing from memory.

When we spend most of our time looking at the page, we try to make what we have drawn so far "make sense" with sneaky embellishments that are not true to life and get in the way later on.

It's a good idea to look at your subject at least 80% of the time while you are drawing. This exercise will help you to practise... by looking at your subject 100% of the time! This practice is called "blind contour drawing". Although you may feel silly as you begin, stick with it – it can really shift how you sense and see while drawing.

Position your paper so the edges are choppy and interesting.

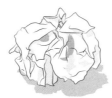 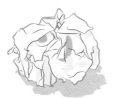

Just draw the contours to begin with.

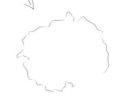 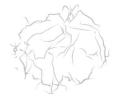

Don't expect the results to be anywhere near perfect! This exercise is all about the process.

Tear out a page from this book (perhaps one that you weren't particularly pleased with). Scrunch up the torn paper and place it about 70 cm / 28 in. away on the table in front of you.

Explore the paper with your eyes, noticing the shapes and textures created by the light as it touches it.

Play with how the piece of paper is sitting, turn it over, rotate it and alter its shape until its natural patterns appear interesting and dynamic.

Without looking down at the page, begin to draw the unique contours of the piece of paper. Aim to copy what your eye is seeing. You are "tracing" the edge of your subject onto the page.

Once you have drawn all the way around the edge of the piece of paper, **still without looking down at the page**, begin to draw the patterns of lines within it.

Remember you are not looking at a piece of paper; you are looking at a bundle of lines and shadows that your mind is labelling "scrunched up paper".

As you shift from verbal to visual interpretation, you may notice a natural quietening of the mind. A lowering of the volume of inner chatter.

NEGATIVE TO POSITIVE

The upside-down exercise stopped us from seeing the symbol, the grid stopped us seeing the "whole" and contour drawing made us see the tiny details of the outline and focus our attention on the subject while drawing.

Drawing the negative space in and around the subject is another way of drawing the edge and avoiding seeing the symbol.

Take a look at the chess pieces on the left. Can you see the yogi hidden in the negative space? It requires a subtle shift in perspective to see her. In the following exercise we are attempting to see the shapes made by the overlapping elements of a houseplant as the foreground instead of the background. By drawing these shapes instead of the houseplant, we bypass the left brain's attempts to help us by labelling it "leaf", "stalk", and so on. The shapes we are drawing don't have names... so they're easy to draw!

For this exercise you will need a houseplant or a vase filled with flowers to use as your subject.

Place your houseplant on the table in front of you and begin to study it.

Notice the shapes of negative space created by the overlapping leaves.

One at a time, draw the shapes of the negative space.

Remember to draw one line at a time. Drawing teaches us patience. Accuracy takes time.

Once you have completed the internal shapes, see if you can draw the negative space that is around the plant.

Now that you have the shape of your plant, feel free to add more detail!

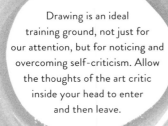

Drawing is an ideal training ground, not just for our attention, but for noticing and overcoming self-criticism. Allow the thoughts of the art critic inside your head to enter and then leave.

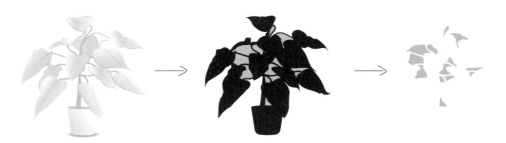

We naturally see our subject as the foreground and ignore background elements.

We can shift our perspective to learn to see the negative space between objects.

Drawing the negative space bypasses seeing the labels we naturally project.

"The flower is made of non-flower elements.

We can describe the flower as being full of everything.

There is nothing that is not present in the flower.

We see sunshine, we see the rain, we see clouds, we see the earth, and we also see time and space in the flower. (...)

The whole cosmos has come together in order to help the flower manifest herself.

The flower is full of everything except one thing: a separate self, a separate identity."

Thích Nhất Hạnh

BECOMING ONE WITH THE SUBJECT

Drawing is a uniquely meditative activity. We enter a flowing state of concentration as we use our bodies and minds to interpret the world around us. When translating an impression from your vision into art on the page you are no longer separate from the object of your perception. You are a fluid part of a much larger process. The image is flowing from the physical, through your consciousness and back out onto the paper.

When you achieve this state, when your mind is devoid of verbal interference, descriptions and labels, your perception is clear. When you are absorbed in your subject, you become a flawless mirror in which the universe is reflecting itself with honesty and without judgements.

For a few moments you are one with the object of your focus.

In yoga, the highest state one can achieve is *"Samadhi"* or oneness with the object of one's perception. In this state the meditator loses their sense of self, transcending their mental separation from the world and experiencing the interconnectedness of all things. I can't think of a faster and more rewarding shortcut than drawing nature from life.

Take a walk through your local park, choose a stationary subject, perhaps a tree, or a flower that you find particularly beautiful. Find a peaceful place to sit and observe.

Notice your mind trying to help by describing the subject: "stem", "leaves", "flower", "branches". Pay attention to how your mind groups the elements as one visual subject. Allow these words to pass through your awareness and leave.

Now allow your focus to shift from the verbal to the visual as we have practised over the last few pages. Begin to notice the textures created by the interplay of light and dark. Take in the edges of your subject, its contours and the negative space in and around it – begin to draw.

Pick a few details from your surroundings and draw them into this grid. Perhaps some patterns in the bark of a tree or an interesting layout of stones. By drawing details alone we avoid seeing the whole, we stop seeing the symbol and experience reality directly.

 Complete these lotus patterns with flowing breaths.
Each line consists of at least 25 breaths – roughly five minutes.

WORD TO THE WISE

It's an important skill to be able to distinguish and attain balance between verbal and visual ways of thinking. To be in touch with both analytical and intuitive ways of interpreting the world.

We've focused heavily on training our attention toward our immediate experience, but thinking is far from useless.

Words are like colours painted onto the canvas of your mind. They are powerful organizational tools. We can take our experiences, past and present, and use them to create new ideas and communicate them to other people.

Each word you hear has a ripple effect on your subconscious, pulling on memories and other thought symbols. Used wisely they can prime us for positive ways of thinking.

Concentrate on your breathing as you trace these breath-drawings.

Let each word "fall into" your heart as you breathe and draw, as though it is falling into a deep well.

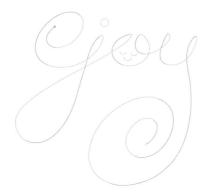

*To feel the full power of words priming your subconscious, try the guided "yoga nidra" at **drawbreath.com***

Mantras are positive affirmations or words thought to have special power or significance, repeated aloud or silently in your head for a specific effect.

This meditative technique appears across many world religions and spiritual practices. Even Christian prayer could be said to be a form of mantra. Not only can the repeated words take up mental space that might otherwise be used for rumination; the right choice of words sends ripples of positive meaning deep into the subconscious, while simultaneously giving us an object of focus on which to practise concentration.

Write yourself a simple mantra below and practise repeating it out loud or silently in your own head.

It can be as personal as a goal or an affirmation, or as innocuous as the shipping forecast!

If you can't think of your own, practise by using the Buddhist mantra *"Om mani padme hum"*, sometimes translated as "the jewel is in the lotus" (wisdom is the path to enlightenment).

Even when we are dressed from head to toe, we rarely notice the sensations caused by our clothes. For most of the day we are offered the soft sensations of garments moving across our bodies, keeping us warm and granting us protection from the world. Yet we are almost never conscious of them until we are prompted or when something feels "wrong". Now that I have mentioned these sensations, you may be noticing them more readily; the feel of your shirt moving across your chest as you breathe, or your glasses resting comfortably on your nose. It's interesting that we so easily notice what was there all along when we're prompted, yet we can take it for granted the rest of the time. This doesn't just apply to sensory feedback.

Just as we don't notice our clothes, our experience of "luck" often needs to be encouraged for us to truly appreciate it. Almost everyone has something that they can feel lucky about.

Luck is never an objective thing; it's not a *fact*. It's subjective, a point of view – a way of interpreting the things around you.

Being lucky is no use unless you *feel* lucky. The luckier you feel, the luckier you are. Not the other way around!

So much of mental life is geared toward problem solving. The mind is designed to solve problems; it needs to find problems to solve. It actively looks for them. But when you proactively use your mind to appreciate your life, your way of experiencing the world changes. Once you notice a few things that you feel grateful for, your world looks very different. It also *feels* different as your body responds to your mind's interpretation of the world as safe and fair, worthwhile and valuable, with balanced physiological responses. It's no surprise that optimists live longer[28]... Lucky them!

Practising gratitude is good for our bodies and minds, and that's something we can all be grateful for.

Gratitude is good for your health (thankfully)

DO YOU FEEL LUCKY?

Draw some things in your life that you feel grateful for in the boxes on this page.

Include doodles of special people, objects with meaning or memories that matter a great deal to you.

How often do you make time to appreciate these things?

Meditate on each of these as you draw. Take your time.

Notice any changes in your mood or your body as you call these things to mind.

A breathtaking thought

If you cannot think of something to feel grateful for, feel grateful for this chance to be alive and breathing. Truly appreciate your next breath.

A breath isn't something you take. A gift cannot be taken; it can only be received.

INTERBEING

A whirlpool visible on the surface of the ocean is not separate from the water, it is made of the water. It is a pattern made by the water, with water flowing constantly in and out. The water that makes the whirlpool was there before the whirlpool, and it will be there after.

The whirlpool is only ever different from the ocean in an abstract sense. Once we label it "whirlpool" in our heads, we begin to see the whirlpool as "object" and the ocean as "background".

The separation exists only in our minds.

Our minds are adapted to notice, label and categorize patterns as concepts. This is crucial for our ability to interact with our environment, communicate with one another and think creatively. But it also stops us from experiencing reality directly. Our reductive concepts *about* reality are in the way.

We are patterns on the surface of the universe. We are made of energy, we are patterns of energy. Energy flows in and out of us. It was there before us and it will be there after. We see ourselves as the "subject" and the rest of the universe as "background", but really, we are no more separate from the universe than the whirlpool is from the ocean.

As you trace the guided whirlpool, visualize a single oxygen molecule flowing into you, becoming part of you, part of your pattern, energizing and strengthening you, and then flowing out.

At what point does the oxygen start, and stop, being "you"?

Becoming "one with the universe" isn't complicated or mysterious.

It simply means realizing that you are only separate from *everything in* the universe on an abstract, linguistic level.

We are projecting the illusion of separateness, of "self" and "other", with our minds, and reinforcing it every time we use the word "I".

By focusing on the breath flowing through us, we can know and experience ourselves as inseparable from the world around us.

You are a dynamic, living pattern in an ever-moving, and much larger, picture.

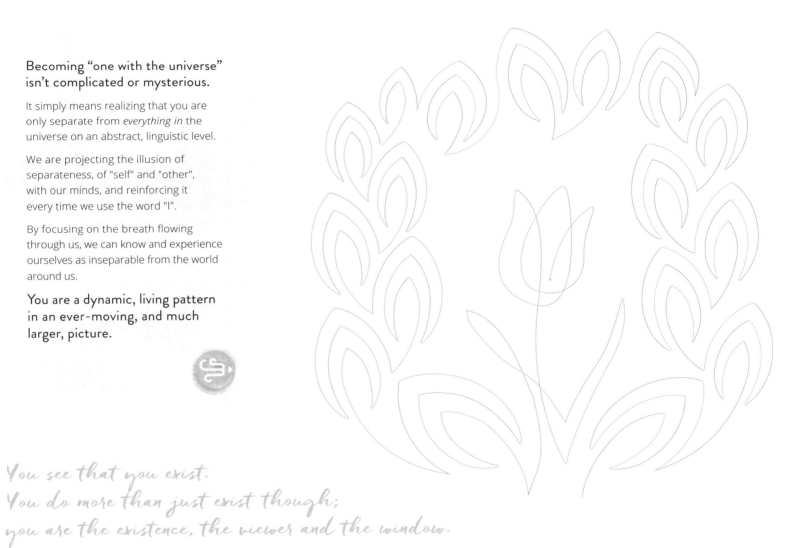

You see that you exist.
You do more than just exist though;
you are the existence, the viewer and the window.

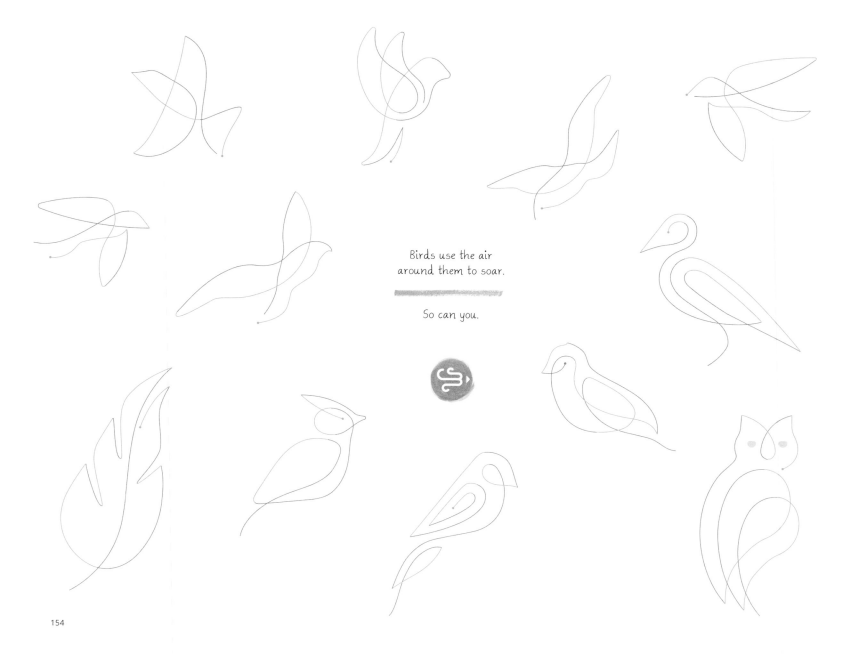

Birds use the air
around them to soar.

So can you.

EXAMPLES OF OTHER PEOPLE'S WORK FROM THE BOOK...

There's no "right" way to "*draw breath*". People's interpretations of the instructions featured in this book vary widely. Finding what is right for you, or, in other words, what helps you to connect to and notice your breath from one moment to the next, is more important than the resulting image looking perfect or even being accurate.

All of the practices in *Draw Breath* are much more about the process than the final result.

I've included the examples on the right so you can see how free-form you can be, and how varied the final results are from person to person.

Have you found the exercises in this book rewarding?

Share your creations with the *Draw Breath* community and inspire others:

#DrawBreathBook

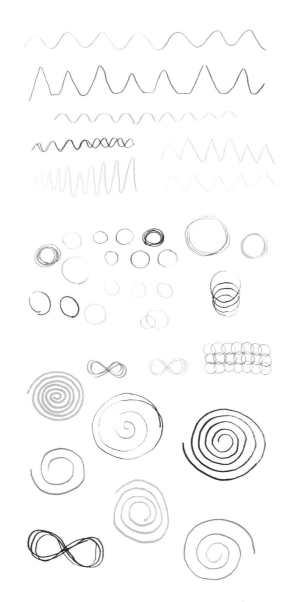

Don't forget that *Draw Breath*'s free-breathing exercises can be done anywhere, anytime.

You don't need the book anymore – just a pencil, some paper and your breath!

These simple, informal meditations are a great way to relax, unwind and mindfully connect your body and mind.

Some people find themselves drawn to one shape in the book, perhaps the spiral or the infinity symbol, that becomes their "go-to" mini meditation. This symbol appears on their notepads and gas bills, a record in the physical world of what occurs in the world of experience.

Which shape are you drawn to?

What animal would you like to see "Draw Breathalized"? What is your patronus? Suggest an animal for me to illustrate using the book's hashtag!

FURTHER READING

I hope you have enjoyed reading *Draw Breath* as much as I enjoyed making it! The following list includes some of the highlights and key influences that I loved reading during my research.

The Breathing Book
Donna Farhi

Drawing on the Right Side of the Brain
Betty Edwards

The Power of Now
Eckhart Tolle

The Healing Power of the Breath
Richard P. Brown and Patricia L. Gerbarg

Just Breathe
Dan Brulé

The Heart of Yoga
T. K. V. Desikachar

Mindfulness
Prof Mark Williams & Dr Danny Penman

Mindfulness for Health
Vidyamala Burch & Dr Danny Penman

Mindfulness for Creativity
Dr Danny Penman

The Open-Focus Brain
Dr Les Fehmi and Jim Robbins

Focus
Daniel Goleman

Asana Pranayama Mudra Bandha
Swami Satyananda Saraswati

The Art of Creative Thinking
Rod Judkins

Full Catastrophe Living
Jon Kabat-Zinn

Mindfulness & the Art of Drawing
Wendy Ann Greenhalgh

Authentic Happiness
Martin Seligman

Thinking, Fast and Slow
Daniel Kahneman

The Way of Zen
Alan Watts

Waking Up
Sam Harris

Check out **LoveYogaLoveLife.org**, a website run by a psychologist and yoga teacher for evidence-based yoga news, classes, meditations and courses in yoga-based health coaching.

APPS

For those interested in exploring biofeedback for breathing, I highly recommend the free **BellyBio** app. This simple app uses clever technology to play beautiful ambient music and wave sounds in response to your breathing to help you achieve depth and rhythm.

There are many useful smartphone apps available for free that allow you to set timers to pace your breath. I recommend experimenting with **xhale breathing**, **Breathe+** and **iBreathe** and seeing which is right for you.

REFERENCES

1   Shannahoff-Khalsa, David S., Michael R. Boyle, and Marcia E. Buebel. "The effects of unilateral forced nostril breathing on cognition." *International Journal of Neuroscience* 57.3–4 (1991): 239–249.

2   Based on an approximation of 32 ml of CO_2 excretion per exhalation.

3   Howland, Robert H. "Vagus nerve stimulation." *Current Behavioral Neuroscience Reports* 1.2 (2014): 64–73.

4   Porges, Stephen W. "Vagal tone: a physiologic marker of stress vulnerability." *Pediatrics* 90.3 (1992): 498–504.

5   Koopman, Frieda A., et al. "Vagus nerve stimulation inhibits cytokine production and attenuates disease severity in rheumatoid arthritis." *Proceedings of the National Academy of Sciences* 113.29 (2016): 8284–8289.

6   Brown, Richard, and Patricia Gerbarg. *The Healing Power of the Breath: Simple techniques to reduce stress and anxiety,* enhance concentration, and balance your emotions. Shambhala Publications, 2012.

7   Streeter, Chris C., et al. "Treatment of major depressive disorder with Iyengar yoga and coherent breathing: a randomized controlled dosing study." *The Journal of Alternative and Complementary Medicine* 23.3 (2017): 201–207.

8   Julien, Claude. "The enigma of Mayer waves: facts and models." *Cardiovascular Research* 70.1 (2006): 12–21.

9   Tawakol, Ahmed, et al. "Relation between resting amygdalar activity and cardiovascular events: a longitudinal and cohort study." *The Lancet* 389.10071 (2017): 834–845.

10 von Zglinicki, Thomas. "Oxidative stress shortens telomeres." *Trends in Biochemical Sciences* 27.7 (2002): 339–344.

11 Tolahunase, Madhuri, Rajesh Sagar and Rima Dada. "Impact of yoga and meditation on cellular aging in apparently healthy individuals: a prospective, open-label single-arm exploratory study." *Oxidative Medicine and Cellular Longevity* 2017 (2017).

12 Calabrese, Pascale, et al. "Cardiorespiratory interactions during resistive load breathing." *American Journal of Physiology-Regulatory, Integrative and Comparative Physiology* 279.6 (2000): R2208–R2213.

13 Twal, Waleed O., Amy E. Wahlquist, and Sundaravadivel Balasubramanian. "Yogic breathing when compared to attention control reduces the levels of pro-inflammatory biomarkers in saliva: a pilot randomized controlled trial." *BMC Complementary and Alternative Medicine* 16.1 (2016): 294.

14 Schulz, André, and Claus Vögele. "Interoception and stress." *Frontiers in Psychology* 6 (2015): 993.

15 Craig, Arthur D. "How do you feel? Interoception: the sense of the physiological condition of the body." *Nature Reviews Neuroscience* 3.8 (2002): 655.

16, 17 Craig, Bud. "How do you feel? Lecture by Bud Craig." Vimeo.com, Medicinska fakulteten vid LiU, 2010, https://vimeo.com/8170544.

18 Killingsworth, Matthew A., and Daniel T. Gilbert. "A wandering mind is an unhappy mind." *Science* 330.6006 (2010): 932–932.

19 Raghunathan, Raj. "How negative is your 'mental chatter'?" *Psychology Today* (2013).

20 Lazar, Sara W., et al. "Meditation experience is associated with increased cortical thickness." *Neuroreport* 16.17 (2005): 1893.

21 Based on the idea that the fovea covers 5% of the retina. Even though peripheral vision accounts for over 90% of visual field only 50% of retinal sensitivity is peripheral (due to density of cones in fovea).

22 Hummel, Friedhelm, and Christian Gerloff. "Larger interregional synchrony is associated with greater behavioral success in a complex sensory integration task in humans." *Cerebral Cortex* 15.5 (2004): 670–678.

23 Provine, Robert R., and Kenneth R. Fischer. "Laughing, smiling, and talking: Relation to sleeping and social context in humans." *Ethology* 83.4 (1989): 295–305.

24 Andrade, Jackie. "What does doodling do?." *Applied Cognitive Psychology: The Official Journal of the Society for Applied Research in Memory and Cognition* 24.1 (2010): 100–106.

25 Gupta, Sharat. "Doodling: The artistry of the roving metaphysical mind." *Journal of Mental Health and Human Behaviour* 21.1 (2016): 16.

26 Kok, Bethany E., et al. "How positive emotions build physical health: perceived positive social connections account for the upward spiral between positive emotions and vagal tone." *Psychological Science* 24.7 (2013): 1123–1132.

27 Kalyani, Bangalore G., et al. "Neurohemodynamic correlates of 'OM' chanting: A pilot functional magnetic resonance imaging study." *International Journal of Yoga* 4.1 (2011): 3.

28 Kim, Eric S., et al. "Optimism and cause-specific mortality: a prospective cohort study." *American Journal of Epidemiology* 185.1 (2017): 21–29.

ABOUT THE AUTHOR

Tom Granger is an author, designer and illustrator based in the UK. He works as a freelance creative consultant for some of the world's most innovative healthcare companies. He has worked extensively for the NHS and for Breathworks, the UK's leading mindfulness teacher training organization. Tom is an enthusiastic meditator and loves all things philosophy, art and yoga.

MORE FROM TOM

Tom also writes humorous, interactive, ironic "self-help" books under the name Tom Devonald. His award-winning works include *The Colouring Book for Goths: The world's most depressing book,* a colouring book designed to be coloured *entirely in black* to help the reader achieve "a demeanour of aloof cynicism"; *The Breakup Journal: Break up without the breakdown*, a surprisingly helpful, light-hearted guide to surviving a split; and finally, *The Love Scrapbook*, an irreverent activity book, perfect for anyone who wants to get creative and make a unique gift for the one they love.

BEYOND THE BOOK

If you have enjoyed this book and found the practices relaxing or rewarding and you'd like to use the techniques as a regular informal meditation (without having to buy a new book every time!), I have made some of the basic patterns available for free for you to print at home. *Please go to DrawBreath.com to find out more*. You will also find additional *guided audio meditations available, absolutely free*. These are perfect for anyone with a budding interest in the themes of this book. Submit your email on the website to be kept in the loop on future *workshops, talks and additions to the world of Draw Breath,* as well as news on the latest innovations and findings in breathwork from around the world.

Follow @DrawBreath on instagram for the latest updates

Visit DrawBreath.com for interesting articles and free activities

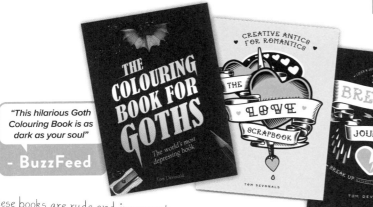

"This hilarious Goth Colouring Book is as dark as your soul"

- BuzzFeed

These books are rude and irreverent. You have been warned!

You can also support *Draw Breath* by purchasing fun and funky art prints like this panda mandala (or "pandala"!).

Head to **DrawBreath.com** and click "shop" to find a print that's right for you!

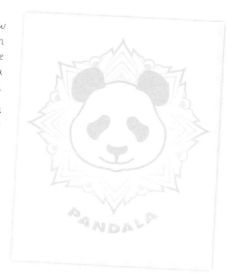

THANK YOU...

... to my **incredible family,** for your unwavering and steadfast support of this utterly bonkers project! In particular, Mum, thank you for your encyclopaedic knowledge of all things yoga and psychology. *Draw Breath* would not have been possible without your input, guidance and brutally honest art direction. Dad, thank you for inspiring me every day with your work ethic and tenacity, and for tolerating the never-ending stream of paper flying out of your printer, (as well as the many psytrance playlist suggestions)! Max, thanks for your firm belief when I was strongly doubting the whole thing! I love you all and am so very lucky to have you as my fam. (So you can all stop fishing for compliments.)

... to **Ione** for sharing much of this journey and for your encouragement, support and boundless enthusiasm for the many forms *Draw Breath* has taken over the years before it got here.

... to **Georgina** and **Saffron** for helping to create the beautiful watercolour textures that appear throughout the book; it wouldn't have looked half as good without your combined, innate artistic spirit and creative flourish.

... to everyone at Summersdale for making this book a reality. Thanks in particular to **Claire** for believing in the fledgling version of the idea, and to **Debbie** and **Lucy** for your expertise and patience in helping nurture it into a fully-fledged book!

... to the many unsuspecting guinea pigs and proof readers along the way, including but not limited to, **Mr and Mrs Harris**. Neil, thank you for every one of our many unintentional, blue-sky-thinking, outdoor, late-night dialectics over the last fifteen years, the sum of which undoubtedly became the seed of this idea.

... to **Anna Black,** your inspiring and rewarding mindful drawing workshop was exactly the confirmation I needed that I wasn't mad for thinking this might be a good idea.

... to **Vidyamala Burch** and the Breathworks team for your sage advice and input on the more mindful and compassionate elements of *Draw Breath*.

... to **Professor Mark Williams** and **Danny Penman** for your invaluable encouragement during the final editing stages.

... to **Patricia Gerbarg** for sharing the sum of your (and **Richard Brown**'s) many years of research with me so clearly in your insightful last-minute edits.

... to **Dan Brulé** for your inspiring works, words and raw-spirited enthusiasm for the project.

... to **Jan** and **Jo** at Mindful Outlook for your excellent 8-week MBSR course.

... to **Agata**, the life-drawing instructor turned qigong master. Your classes came at just the right time! And to the **mystery man** in Whalley Range for the free open-air Tai Chi lessons in Alexandra Park all those summers ago.

... to the inspiringly irreverent creative faculty at King's Macc, **Mr Hiddon**, **Frank Walker** and **Gill Taylor,** for teaching me, through osmosis, that creative mischief is a way of life.

... to the teachers, **Davies**, **Bailey** and **MacDonald**, and the Philosophy faculty at Notts Uni, (particularly **Greg Mason**) for forever conflating the concepts of philosophy and witty repartee in my mind.

... to **Wolf** for giving me my break at The Raft. To **Lee**, **Rich** and **Kev** for showing me the creative ropes. To **Richard**, **Clare**, **Melissa** and **Simon** for the freedom and self-direction of the Run Creative times, (also I broke into your office when you weren't there and used your printer to print the manuscript for this book (sorry not sorry)). To **DMB**, thanks for the kind gift that helped me create many of the illustrations in this book. We'll always have "Ibiza".

... to many *thousands* of passionate and knowledgeable Redditors for unwittingly helping my research over the last few years on the r/art, r/meditation and r/Buddhism forums. (TLDR: I'm thanking everyone).

Finally, to all of the amazing friends, freaks, family and festival revellers from around the world that I have met on this adventure into yoga, qigong, mindfulness, meditation, philosophy and art; thanks for making it so downright... *fun.*

(I'm not just saying all this because gratitude is good for my health...

... honestly!)

Now is
always
beginning

and never
ending

Have you enjoyed this book?
If so, why not write a review on your favourite website?

If you're interested in finding out more about our books,
find us on Facebook at **Summersdale Publishers**
and follow us on Twitter at @Summersdale.

Thanks very much for buying this Summersdale book.
www.summersdale.com

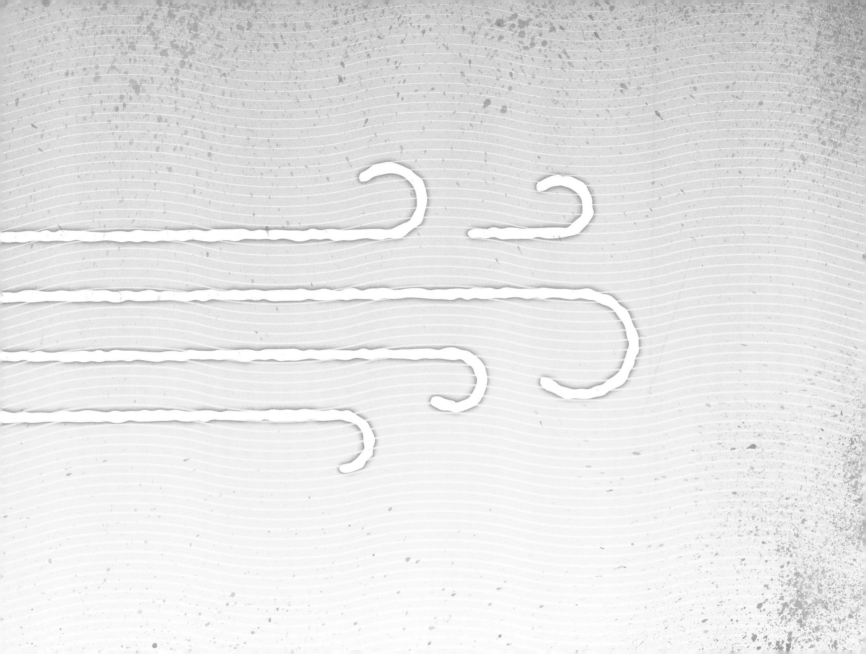

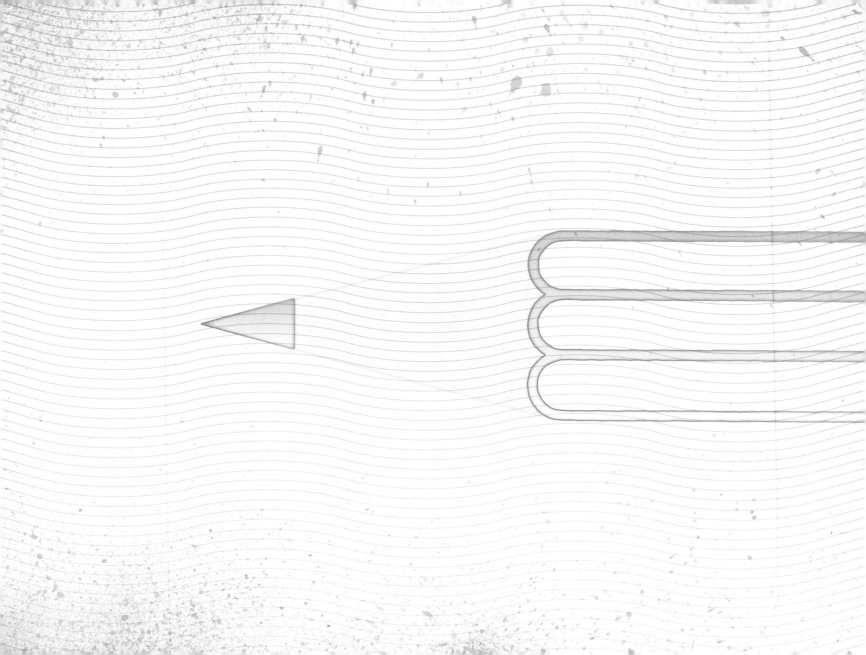